Fibromyalgia

Fibromyalgia

Kim D. Jones and
Janice H. Hoffman

Biographies of Disease
Julie K. Silver, M.D., Series Editor

GREENWOOD PRESS

An Imprint of ABC-CLIO, LLC

A B C **≋** C L I O

Santa Barbara, California • Denver, Colorado • Oxford, England

Library of Congress Cataloging-in-Publication Data
Jones, Kim D.
 Fibromyalgia / Kim D. Jones and Janice H. Hoffman.
   p. cm. — (Biographies of disease)
 Includes bibliographical references and index.
 ISBN 978-0-313-36440-2 (hard copy : alk. paper) — ISBN 978-0-313-36441-9 (ebook)
 1. Fibromyalgia—Popular works. I. Hoffman, Janice H. II. Title.
 RC927.3.J66 2009
 616.7'42—dc22   2009032509

13 12 11 10 9   1 2 3 4 5

This book is also available on the World Wide Web as an eBook.
Visit www.abc-clio.com for details.

ABC-CLIO, LLC
130 Cremona Drive, P.O. Box 1911
Santa Barbara, California 93116-1911

This book is printed on acid-free paper ∞

Manufactured in the United States of America

Contents

Series Foreword

Every disease has a story to tell: about how it started long ago and began to disable or even take the lives of its innocent victims, about the way it hurts us, and about how we are trying to stop it. In this Biographies of Disease series, the authors tell the stories of the diseases that we have come to know and dread.

The stories of these diseases have all of the components that make for great literature. There is incredible drama played out in real-life scenes from the past, present, and future. You'll read about how men and women of science stumbled trying to save the lives of those they aimed to protect. Turn the pages and you'll also learn about the amazing success of those who fought for health and won, often saving thousands of lives in the process.

If you don't want to be a health professional or research scientist now, when you finish this book you may think differently. The men and women in this book are heroes who often risked their own lives to save or improve ours. This is the biography of a disease, but it is also the story of real people who made incredible sacrifices to stop it in its tracks.

Julie K. Silver, M.D.
Assistant Professor, Harvard Medical School
Department of Physical Medicine and Rehabilitation

Preface

This book is written for you, the next generation of scientists, clinicians, advocates, and patients. You will carry scientific discovery to the next level, alleviating suffering for millions around the globe. You will provide rational, compassionate care to people who have been maligned for centuries. You will move legislation forward that will protect jobs and health care for those with fibromyalgia. You may even forward the cause by being a patient with fibromyalgia yourself someday; if this occurs, the knowledge provided in this book may be the key to a more hopeful and less painful tomorrow.

Three decades of objective scientific evidence finally has transitioned from a suspicious set of symptoms into a real diagnosis: fibromyalgia. This book is written as a first edition, because only now has the scientific and medical community come to accept these three critical facts: first, fibromyalgia is a distinct disorder with reproducible, objective abnormalities; second, fibromyalgia has a rigorous diagnostic criteria and is no longer considered a "wastebasket" diagnosis; third, fibromyalgia has myriad effective treatments, including three medications that recently have passed the scrutiny of the Food and Drug Administration and are labeled as specific for fibromyalgia treatment.

The authors provide you with the tools you need to rapidly assimilate new knowledge in your understanding of fibromyalgia. The information is garnered from top health-care journals, our own research, participation in international scientific meetings, and clinical practice. You are provided with original, easy-to-understand art to depict scientifically dense concepts. The book is organized by defining fibromyalgia, clearly explaining its pathophysiology, explaining the clinician's role, discussing the assemblage of an ideal treatment team, explaining the various treatments, detailing other common disorders found in individuals with fibromyalgia, and ending with one young person's personal story and a discussion of self-efficacy for optimal quality of life. All of the stories included throughout the book tell of real people and their lives with fibromyalgia. Commonly used scientific terms are described in lay language in a glossary, and excellent scientific resources can be found in the appendixes and bibliography for further study.

After reading this book you will be prepared to eruditely debate the controversy that still surrounds fibromyalgia and emerge with the confidence to embrace new ideas. All great pioneers in history were encouraged to take the easier path. With health care, as in life, it is often the more challenging path that ultimately provides a richer life with greater achievement. You will be humanity's next pioneers. Enjoy your journey.

Acknowledgments

We wish to acknowledge deep gratitude and professional debt to mentors Robert Bennett, MD, Carol Burckhardt, PhD, and Sharon Clark, PhD. Our sincere thanks to Amy Michelle Wiley who contributed her personal story to Chapter 7; you can read more of her story and her writing on her Web site: www.sparrowsflight.net. Thanks also to Jennifer Hwee and Elizabeth Kwak for their help in preparing our glossary, and to Rachel L. Ward for both her help in locating needed research references and agreeing to be our exercise model. We also extend our thanks to L. Robert Hoffman, our photographer. We acknowledge support from our own fibromyalgia nonprofit organization, the Fibromyalgia Information Foundation (www.myalgia.com). Our further gratitude extends to the international FM research community and all the patients and families who allow us to participate in their care. It is only through their concerted efforts to help conquer this disorder that we are able to provide the information found here.

Introduction

Fibromyalgia (fie-bro-my-AL-gee-a), also referred to as FM, is increasingly being recognized as a real illness. This is a blessing to the many patients whose symptoms were once met with disbelief from health-care professionals and a lack of understanding from family, friends, and coworkers.

Thankfully, today the majority of health-care providers agree FM is a real disorder and the discrimination is finally waning. New clinicians coming out of school have benefited from updated training based on solid research findings; they are knowledgeable about FM, understand the American College of Rheumatology's diagnostic guidelines, and are consequently more likely to correctly diagnose this disorder. FM has specific signs and symptoms that occur together, so it is sometimes referred to as a syndrome. However, a more recent confluence of objective research findings has compelled researchers to label FM a disorder rather than a syndrome. A disorder can be defined as a set of symptoms that are clearly connected by objective, reproducible pathophysiologic changes. A *syndrome* is a broader term used earlier in the understanding of an illness when the underlying abnormalities are not as well understood.

1

What Is Fibromyalgia?

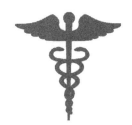

DEFINITION

The hallmark of fibromyalgia (FM) includes the presence of multiple tender points at specific locations over the body, combined with the report of widespread musculoskeletal pain. A good analogy is to consider pain as a radio signal. If the volume control on the receiver is broken and broadcasts only at a greatly amplified sound level, an otherwise normal listening experience will become difficult to tolerate. It is the same type of experience with pain in FM; even typically nonpainful stimuli like a gentle hug can cause discomfort because of pain amplification. This phenomenon is caused in large part by central sensitization, and in fact, many researchers believe the central nervous system is the key factor in the pathology of FM. Like most chronic illnesses, the symptoms of FM extend far beyond the defining criteria. In addition to pain, many patients also report the following co-morbidities (overlapping but separate disorders or symptoms):

- Fatigue
- Muscle and joint stiffness
- Insomnia
- Restless Legs Syndrome (RLS)
- Balance issues, including orthostatic hypotension and dysautonomia
- Headaches, including migraine headaches

- Cognitive lapses
- Raynaud's Phenomenon
- Autoimmune disorders such as Sjögren's Syndrome and rheumatoid arthritis
- Visual, auditory, tactile, and olfactory hypersensitivities
- Irritable bowel and irritable bladder
- Pelvic pain, endometriosis, vulvodynia
- Depression and anxiety disorders
- Temporomandibular joint dysfunction

The symptoms of FM may improve, may worsen, or may be continual, but the disorder is extremely unlikely to completely go away. Periods when symptoms worsen are termed *flares* and are often brought on by physical overexertion or stress. Many people with FM find that, at least some of the time, their illness prevents them from engaging in common everyday activities, such as traveling in a car for prolonged periods and climbing stairs. The disorder can be debilitating and often has a serious impact on family relationships, social friendships, and the ability to stay employed. It is understandable that life satisfaction levels suffer when someone cannot participate in what is considered a normal lifestyle. As is true with most chronic pain conditions, depression and anxiety are a common response to FM symptoms. Unfortunately, some medical providers continue to treat FM as only a psychosomatic disorder despite more and more research confirming FM is, in fact, physical.

There are some further points to remember about this disorder. First, FM is not limited to the musculoskeletal system; research has shown brain and spinal cord involvement. Second, although some persons with FM may first experience primary immune system disorders such as rheumatoid arthritis, systemic lupus erythematosus (SLE), or Sjögren's Syndrome, FM is not in itself an autoimmune disease. Third, we know this disorder is not the same as Chronic Fatigue Immune Dysfunction Syndrome (CFIDS) since people with FM have chemical hallmarks in their spinal column fluid that are not present in CFIDS. Fourth, FM is not a mental illness. Studies have shown there is no higher incidence of mental illness in FM than in many other chronic pain populations.

Overall, it is important to remember that FM is not a catchall diagnosis; it is a chronic, nondegenerative, noninflammatory disorder with an accepted diagnostic criteria.

GLOBAL STATISTICS AND ECONOMIC RESULTS

Approximately 15 million persons in the United States have been diagnosed with FM. It can occur at any point in life but is most commonly diagnosed in middle age. The disorder strikes men, women, and children of all races, although women are diagnosed with FM eight to nine times more often than men. That ratio may change since many returning Gulf War veterans who experienced the chronic stress of being in war and known chemical and toxin exposure are exhibiting symptoms similar to, and which in fact may be, FM.

Since the 1990 College of Rheumatology classification criteria for FM was established, epidemiological studies estimate that the disorder occurs from 1.3 percent to 7.3 percent in the population worldwide. At least fifteen different countries have recorded criteria-based cases of FM, indicating that it is not limited to industrialized countries, and further, affects people of all ages, races, and ethnicities. Despite the outward appearance of normality, persons with this disorder often have difficulty staying in the workforce, and a downward spiral toward work disability is not uncommon. This is especially the case for medically undertreated persons and those who experience many of the overlapping co-morbidities of FM. Approximately 16 percent of FM-diagnosed U.S. citizens receive Social Security benefits, compared to 2.2 percent of the general U.S. population. FM also represents a liability to medical systems in the United States and worldwide. The direct cost of FM medical care in the United States alone is $20 billion annually and the average rate of medical services in the United States for each patient nears $10,000 yearly.

HISTORY

Spinal Irritation is characterized by multiple tender spots distributed over the female body, probably caused by sexual excess. . . . leeches to the inside of the nostrils are remarkably efficacious. . . .

—William A. Hammond, Spinal Irritation, 1886

Many would argue that throughout history the medical ailments suffered mainly by women have been met with medical arrogance and disrespect. FM is no different, as the above quote so well demonstrates. FM is an ancient disorder, with a long history of medical speculation as to its source, contributing factors, and potential treatments. Medical descriptions of symptoms indicating FM can be found dating back to the sixteenth century.

The differences between rheumatic conditions involving joint deformity, termed *articular rheumatism*, and painful but nondeforming muscular rheumatism were recorded at that time. In the early to mid-1800s, a surgeon named William Balfour from Edinburgh, Scotland, and later the physician François Valleix in Paris, independently described unusually painful areas in patients with muscular rheumatism that produced shooting pain when palpated. *Fibrositis* was the term that preceded fibromyalgia. It first came into use in 1904 when English neurologist Sir William Gowers wrote a medical paper on low back pain. He speculated that low back tenderness was due to inflammatory changes in muscle fiber tissue and discussed for the first time the concept of pain amplification, as well as the possible contribution of disrupted sleep and fatigue to diffuse rheumatic muscle pain. However, subsequent studies of muscle biopsies failed to find traditional indications of inflammation, and the term *fibrositis* was then considered a misnomer. At the turn of the twentieth century, physician Sir William Osler coined the term *myalgia* and speculated that the pain of muscular rheumatism involved "neuralgia of the sensory nerves of the muscles." World War II saw an increase in the diagnosis of fibrositis in British soldiers, with 70 percent of all rheumatic patients in British army hospitals diagnosed with the condition.

Over time, the terms *fibrositis*, *fibromyositis*, *muscular rheumatism*, and even "tender lady syndrome" have all been used to describe this disorder. In 1973 the researcher Philip Hench first introduced the term *fibromyalgia*, which more accurately describes the symptoms. This current term is referenced by the following medical root words: *fibra* (Latin for fiber), *myo* (Greek for muscle), and *algos* (Greek for pain). Researchers such as Muhammad B. Yunus, Robert M. Bennett, I. Jon Russell, and others, seeking to clearly define FM in the 1980s, proposed the need for a unified classification system. In 1990, following a rigorous multisite research study, the American College of Rheumatology published a formal "Criteria for the Classification of Fibromyalgia." The American Medical Association recognized FM as a true illness and as a major cause of disability in 1987; the World Health Organization followed with the same recognition in 1992.

2

Diagnosing the Disorder

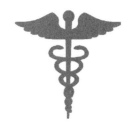

FM rarely occurs out of the blue. Like most chronic illnesses, FM is thought to occur when an environmental trigger overcomes a genetically predisposed individual. For example, people genetically predisposed to lung cancer may experience that illness when exposed to certain pollutants such as cigarette smoke, a known environmental trigger. Following are five real-life presentations of FM from clinical practice. Notice how they are all different in terms of age, gender, ethnicity, symptom severity, disease progression, and possible trigger.

1) Juanita is a 58-year-old Hispanic female homemaker who has a six-year history of increasing aches and pains. She also complains of fatigue and feeling unrefreshed in the morning despite being in bed for nine to ten hours. In the past few months she has noticed it hurts when her husband hugs her or her grandchildren playfully tug on her arms. She denies any accidents, surgery, medications, or illnesses that preceded the onset of her symptoms. She is concerned that she may be getting rheumatism like her mother and grandmother had.

2) Jim is a 36-year-old Caucasian male sales representative with a four-year history of widespread migratory pain that always includes his neck and shoulders. Initially, he attributed the pain to playing competitive racquetball, but he hasn't played now in more than a year, yet has seen no improvement in his

pain symptoms. He has seen multiple providers and had negative imaging studies of his neck, upper back, and both shoulders. He has had no relief from NSAIDs, acetaminophen, massage, or acupuncture. His pain seems to be getting worse and now interferes with his ability to talk on the phone while driving (shoulder to ear), to type at his computer keyboard for more than one hour, and to endure the extended seating required to drive or fly to sales meetings. He continues to work sixty hours per week and "push through the pain." He is concerned that he may have a more serious underlying disease, specifically cancer, since his pain has spread to his entire body during the past six months.

3) Leslie is a 21-year-old Caucasian female college student who was in her usual excellent state of health until six months ago when she was involved in a minor motor vehicle accident. She was diagnosed with whiplash and despite extensive physical therapy, NSAIDs, and faithfully wearing the soft collar her provider prescribed, she has not improved. In fact, over the past three months, her pain has extended to her upper arms, lower back, and hips. Concurrently, her sleep has become increasingly fragmented, and she wakes up several times at night, often unable to return to sleep. Her clinician has been treating her for depression due to her poor sleep and her ongoing concern about her health. The antidepressant medication is not helping her pain, mood, or sleep, and she is worried she may need to drop out of school. Additionally, she feels out of control regarding her health and well-being and wonders why she feels like someone sixty years old.

4) Rachel is a 40-year-old African American female college professor and mother of two. She has complained of pain over most of her body for one year. She had a sudden onset of insomnia after the birth of her first child ten years earlier and has tried multiple over-the-counter sleep medications. Over time she also has tried a dozen different nonmedical therapies from complementary and alternative providers, with no relief from the insomnia or pain. Her medical doctor doesn't believe in the long-term use of sleep or pain medication unless a patient's diagnosis is terminal. She has arrived as a new clinic patient today because "whatever I have is getting worse." Specifically, she has started experiencing gut pain with changes in stool, bladder burning, pain on urination, and headaches that are increasing in frequency and severity.

5) Junko is a 62-year-old Asian female artist who was in her usual excellent state of health until six months ago when she contracted "the flu that never went away." She complains of overwhelming fatigue, has difficulty concentrating, and experiences mild, but always present, pain in her low back, hips, and shoulders. Her symptoms are interfering with her ability to paint or work with her arms held above her shoulders for more than a couple of minutes. She has not improved with antibiotics, antiviral medications, or even steroids. Her routine and autoimmune blood tests are all normal. She is concerned she may

have lupus or multiple sclerosis despite a negative MRI scan and cerebral spinal fluid analysis.

THE CLINICIAN'S ROLE

How would a clinician who suspects FM diagnose a patient? First, a thorough medical history would be taken and questions would be asked about typical FM symptoms. Lab reports, X-rays, and summary letters written by previous specialists such as neurologists, psychiatrists, or endocrinologists would also be requested for review, and the clinician would seek to rule out other diseases that mimic FM. The patient would be asked to complete a Body Pain Diagram (a body outline drawing that the patient shades in to help the clinician visualize which areas have hurt for most days of the week over the past three months). This is analyzed by the clinician to ensure pain has indeed occurred in at least three out of four quadrants of the body, with the inclusion of some part of the spine. The four quadrants are located above the waist, below the waist, left of midline, and right of midline.

Next, the clinician completes a physical examination focusing primarily on the musculoskeletal and neurological system, which would include a Tender Point Survey. This survey is a notation of pain response to careful palpation of specific body locations using a light compression of 4 kg. Other non-FM peripheral pain generators such as bursitis, tendonitis, plantar fasciitis, and osteoarthritis would be reviewed as well. A careful review of the small joints of the hands and feet should reveal those areas to be free from the inflammation or joint degeneration that occurs in various kinds of inflammatory arthritis but not in FM. Finally, the provider would check for possible symptoms of certain other overlapping conditions that do sometimes appear alongside FM.

The eighteen tender-point locations include the following nine bilateral muscle locations:

- Cervical: (front neck area)
- Second rib: (front chest area)
- Occiput: (back of the neck)
- Trapezius: (back shoulder area)
- Supraspinatus: (shoulder blade area)
- Lateral epicondyle: (elbow)
- Gluteal: (buttock)
- Greater trochanter: (hip)
- Vastus medialis: (inner knee)

The case scenarios earlier represent five very common clinical presentations of FM. Note that Jim, Juanita, and Rachel describe the gradual onset of localized to

Tender Point Locations Anterior View

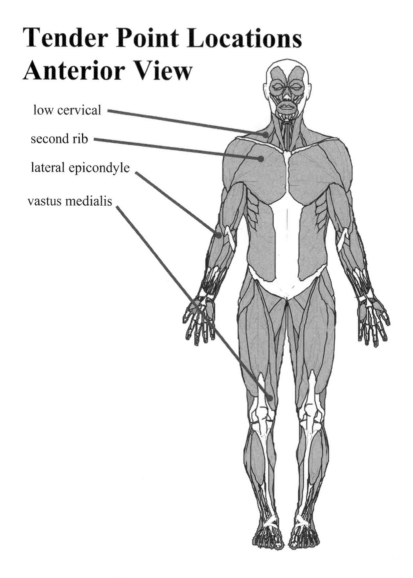

low cervical

second rib

lateral epicondyle

vastus medialis

widespread pain, with varying degrees of fatigue and disrupted sleep. However, Leslie's pain started suddenly after a whiplash-type injury, whereas a virus might have been the trigger for Junko's symptoms. Despite the different presentations, varying symptoms, and different probable triggers, all five of these patients were found to have FM and no other primary medical disease. Once an accurate diagnosis was made, these patients were offered a step-wise recovery plan that included pharmacologic and nonpharmacologic treatments designed to reduce the severity of symptoms, help restore physical functioning, and improve quality of life.

Tender Point Locations Posterior View

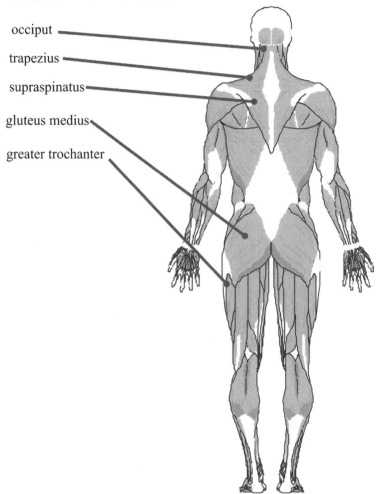

occiput

trapezius

supraspinatus

gluteus medius

greater trochanter

SYMPTOMS AND DIAGNOSIS

As seen, FM symptoms can vary widely between patients. One person's quality of life might be most altered by unremitting pain, whereas a second person may suffer mainly from deep fatigue. Still others might find themselves confronted with anxiety and panic attacks that limit their confidence to travel or work outside the home. Those most severely affected by FM may struggle with all of these symptoms and further co-morbidities.

Additionally, the severity range of FM symptoms is quite unpredictable. Making a comparison with the chronic illness diabetes, a patient might do everything they should by following the correct diet, exercising as advised, carefully controlling blood sugar, and taking prescribed medication. Yet they may still experience a poor outcome, with the eventual loss of a leg or eye, or experience a heart attack, or undergo kidney failure. However, others with the same form of diabetes who make the same medical and lifestyle choices will not suffer the same outcome. In the same way, some FM patients, through no fault of their own, are severely affected by their disorder whereas others will have an easier path. Some researchers have suggested there may be more than one type of FM, distinguishable by differing severity and symptoms. This hypothesis of subtypes is understandable. Consider that it would be no different from past research discovering there was more than one type of cancer, or that there were several kinds of diabetes or dyslipidemias (cholesterol and triglyceride problems in the blood). Scientists are currently looking for laboratory markers to more clearly define potential subtypes in the belief this will eventually lead to more specific and effective treatments.

Pain in FM might be experienced as aching, stabbing, burning, numbness, or all of the above at different times. People with FM often describe their muscles as feeling torn, exhausted, or overworked. They may also feel muscles twitch or even spasm. Sometimes the pain is felt deep in muscles and bones, while at other times it is located more toward the surface of the body. Most patients say their pain is always present, although the severity will wax and wane at different times throughout the day, with weather changes, and after stress or exertion. Back pain is the most common location of pain in FM. It is the job of the clinician to rule out any other causes of back pain and to recommend repair for pain that can be helped by regional anesthesia or surgical procedures. Stiffness is one of the least understood symptoms, although most persons with FM describe painful body stiffness first thing in the morning or after extended periods of stillness. Patients sometimes complain of stiffness with the added sensation of swollen joints, although actual synovitis (an abnormal fluid collection in joints) is not a part of FM, and so the true cause would need to be investigated.

Most everyone can recall the last time they felt exhausted from a bad flu or suffered from fatigue after a case of jet lag. The difference for FM patients is that they feel a similar kind of fatigue and exhaustion that will come and go for the rest of their lives. While FM is more common than Chronic Fatigue Immune Dysfunction Syndrome (CFIDS), an overlap does exist, with some patients diagnosed with both disorders. Persons with CFIDS experience an unremitting form of fatigue that is unrelieved by rest and not known to be caused by another medical explanation.

Nonrefreshing sleep or insomnia also can create fatigue in FM. In nonrefreshing sleep, people report they sleep for 10-plus hours but wake up feeling unrefreshed, or as one patient put it, "feeling like I've been run over by a Mack truck." Other people with fatigue in FM have insomnia. Insomnia can include difficulty falling asleep, difficulty staying asleep, or early morning waking. All of these sleep disruptions are either caused by, or adversely affect, the body's hormonal and nervous system functioning. Multiple sleep studies consistently have demonstrated abnormalities in the sleep architecture of people with FM. It can be challenging for clinicians to correctly differentiate the fatigue of FM from a diagnosis of general muscle weakness. True muscle weakness appears in neurological diseases such as multiple sclerosis (also called MS, a condition in which the immune system attacks the central nervous system, leading to a loss of normal nerve structure and function). It involves an inability in muscle endurance that will cancel movement. Muscle fatigue in FM is different because a person with FM can continue to move if they must although that movement will be increasingly painful. And while the muscles feel painful, all major muscles, muscle reflexes, and muscle metabolism remain normal; in other words, the muscle-nerve connections do not degenerate in FM.

At any given time 30 percent of those diagnosed with FM are thought to be depressed, and 60 percent have experienced depression at some point in the past. Though debate continues over whether mood disorders precipitate FM, or vice versa, it remains true that mood disorders are common in FM. It is essential to good quality of life that patients receive adequate pharmacologic or nonpharmacologic treatment. Specific criteria are used to diagnose various mood problems, and treatment will vary with the diagnosis. Difficulty thinking clearly or multitasking is another symptom recently recognized in FM. Sometimes called fibro-fog, difficulty with cognition is reported to be one of the most distressing symptoms of FM. People also report difficulty with short-term recall tasks such as remembering names or completing tasks. This is not a symptom of lowered IQ or dementia. Enough patients with FM have been seen by the medical community that, if a link did exist between FM and IQ or dementia, clinicians would have realized and reported it years ago.

Clinicians and patients report balance impairment in FM. Symptoms of poor balance include being accident prone, feeling lightheaded, and experiencing falls. Balance involves more than simple muscle strength. Inadequate signals from proprioception (feedback of relative body position) in muscles and tendons, visual cues, vestibular cues (inner ear signals), and delayed reaction time all can play a part in injury. Researchers continue to look into the reasons for balance problems in this disorder. Recent studies hypothesize that the peripheral and/or central mechanisms of postural control are being affected. Further study will help identify the relative contributions of neural and musculoskeletal impairments to postural stability and help develop interventions to minimize these impairments.

In 1990, based on a multisite research study, the American College of Rheumatology adopted the classification criteria for FM. The research study compared patients with FM to people with other chronic pain conditions, such as lupus and rheumatoid arthritis, and then considered the symptom findings in FM against people with no known disease (called healthy controls). In addition to a body pain diagram and Tender Point Survey exam, all research subjects completed questionnaires about many other symptoms associated with FM. Interestingly, it was the combination of widespread pain on the body diagram and at least eleven of eighteen tender points on the physical exam that differentiated the FM patients from not only the healthy controls but those with other pain conditions.

While these criteria originally were developed to ensure that FM patients in research studies were as similar as possible, the classification criteria has migrated into the clinical arena and is considered the current gold standard for diagnosing FM in a clinical setting. The 1990 ACR diagnosis criteria may change in the future when laboratory markers develop that are inexpensive and easy to use in a clinic setting. Examples of markers in other diagnoses include using a sphygmomanometer for determining high blood pressure and glucose testing to detect diabetes. The current objective laboratory markers in FM are not so easily measured in a health-care clinic setting. They require a combination of functional brain imaging with evoked pain, cerebral spinal fluid analyses taken at rest, blood tests taken during the stress of acute exercise, overnight laboratory-based sleep studies, and resting heart rate variability monitoring. In addition to being burdensome and time consuming for the patient, third-party payers generally do not reimburse for these tests to make a diagnosis of FM. More often, these selected tests are reimbursed when a clinician is ruling out a secondary diagnosis in FM, like sleep apnea or multiple sclerosis.

Regarding tender point exams, it is possible that the female-to-male gender discrepancy seen in FM diagnosis could be artificially inflated due to the 4 kg of pressure used in Tender Point Survey criteria. The pain threshold of manual palpation criteria established in 1990 by the ACR may need to be moved to a higher level for men due to gender differences in musculature. As a greater number of men return from war service with widespread pain and become candidates for a diagnosis of FM, perhaps a revision of current criteria will take place. In summary, pain can be seen objectively in a variety of research tests and consequently, our understanding of chronic pain, including FM, is soaring.

3

Those at Risk

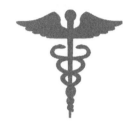

KNOWN RISK FACTORS AND CAUSATION HYPOTHESES

In most chronic illnesses a single lead cause eludes researchers, and FM is no different. However, scientists continue to develop a number of hypotheses about who may develop this disorder and why based on good objective evidence. Along with demographic studies and recorded clinical observations that highlight known risk factors, causation hypotheses are helpful in indicating further possible risk. Both known and suspected risk factors include: gender, age, genetics, viral infection, stress, nervous system malfunctioning, sleep disturbances, and hormonal discrepancies.

Gender, Age, and Genetics

The two greatest known risk factors for FM appear to be a family history of the disease and being female. In fact, two recent studies have revealed that FM in a first-degree female relative is the greatest predictor of developing FM. No one knows why more women are diagnosed with FM than men. Various studies based on prevalence data show that women are seven to nine times more likely to have fibromyalgia than men and that the female peak age for diagnosis is during the childbearing years. This has led researchers to suspect that either childbirth or menopause might be triggers for some women. However, there are no data to support the idea that gender-specific hormones such as estrogen, progesterone, or testosterone are linked to the development of the disorder.

FM is found in all age ranges from children to the frail elderly. Research funded by the National Institutes of Health has begun to find out more about FM in both of these age spans. One study found that one-quarter of adult FM patients report their symptoms started before fifteen years of age. Other studies have shown that the disorder's principal symptoms are the same for children as for adults, although children have more commonly reported nighttime growing pains, pain in extremities, poor sleep, and difficulty keeping up with their peers in athletic endeavors. In contrast, children have reported less low back pain, hand pain, or symptom changes associated with mood or weather. Indeed, pain is not one of the primary complaints in children with FM. This is likely because young children have a hard time knowing their pain isn't normal. Claudia Marek, author of *The First Year—Fibromyalgia*, interviewed a group of children and was amazed to discover 50 percent of her interviewees thought everyone they knew had pain but that other children were simply braver and better at coping with it than they were. Consequently, they were unwilling to verbalize their distress to others. In fact, for many children with FM, the pain they experience is "normal" to them. Since they have not experienced life without the disorder, they cannot distinguish their symptoms as unusual. FM can be quite severe in childhood. Similar steps to those used for diagnosing FM in adults are used by pediatric providers: a medical history is taken, other possible causes for the symptoms are ruled out, and a Tender Point Survey is performed. Children and adolescents with FM may report as few as five tender points. As discussed earlier, this can be because their experience of normal pain is skewed and leads to an underestimation of pressure pain severity during the test.

Children with FM are often misdiagnosed at first with mood disorders or other conditions, and it is not unusual for families seeking help for their children to have difficult experiences before receiving the correct diagnosis. Beyond the same discounting of symptoms adults with FM have received from the medical community in the past, some parents report they were unjustly accused of poor parenting by encouraging their child toward an imaginary disability, or even of inventing illness in a bid for the parents to receive heightened attention. Sometimes it is the cognitive problems experienced with FM that will first alert parents to seek medical help for their child. When this happens the more recognized learning disorders such as dyslexia or attention deficit disorder (ADD) are often explored and ruled out before finding the correct diagnosis. One discernable difference between children with dyslexia or other learning difficulties and those with FM is that those with learning difficulties will have a consistent struggle to perform certain tasks, whereas a young student who has no difficulty concentrating on schoolwork one day, but struggles on other days, may be displaying the fibro-fog of FM.

On the other end of the age spectrum, older adults bear the greatest burden of FM. One study found that only 9 percent of consecutively enrolled older adults tested for FM had previously received the diagnosis. Other painful conditions that come with aging may be the culprit. As an example, multiple surgeries, especially back and pelvic or abdominal surgeries, are associated as triggers for FM, and so age itself may also be a trigger for FM. Alternately, one of the greatest risks for elderly patients who have been diagnosed with FM is that other diseases may be blamed on FM and thereby overlooked. For example, cardiac chest pain can be misdiagnosed as tender-point chest pain by either the patient or the clinician, while widespread pain from metastatic (spreading) cancer or the typical fatigue of undetected hypothyroidism (low thyroid disease) or anemia may be misinterpreted as the pain and fatigue of FM. Back pain with numbness, tingling, or radiating to the hips and legs may be neurologic in nature and not due to FM. Severe hip osteoarthritis (degenerating joint inflammation) is often overlooked in FM because of an older patient's longstanding pain, or may be attributed to the lessening mobility and de-conditioning associated with normal aging. Autoimmune diseases such as polymyalgia rheumatica (PMR, an inflammatory condition) in persons older than 50 can also be misdiagnosed as FM despite a simple blood test called a sedimentation rate that could easily differentiate the two. This type of searching beyond the explanation of FM pain is critical; for example, undiagnosed PMR can sometimes progress to irreversible blindness.

There is a high aggregation of FM in families and so genetics undoubtedly play a part in the development of FM. Two genes in particular seem to be implicated; the COMT gene (short for the Catechol-O-methyl transferase gene associated with certain reductions of dopamine) and the serotonin transporter gene repeatedly have been found to be more common in people with FM than in the general population. Other genes in the dopamine and catecholamine transport systems also may have a role. It is important to note that a family history of FM can include more than genetics. Family environment does need to be taken into account as well. Possible environmental factors that may contribute to FM would include long-term poor diet and lack of regular medical attention associated with poverty, sedentary lifestyle, physical trauma, emotional trauma, and cigarette smoking.

Viruses

Viruses are found wherever life is present. First discovered in 1899, a virus (Latin for poison or toxin) is a microscopic infectious agent. They are about 100 times smaller than bacteria and are acellular (cannot grow through cell division), so they cannot self-reproduce. Instead, they invade and use the cells of each host to produce multiple copies of themselves. A virus can initiate a cascade of abnormal changes in the body, and in genetically susceptible individuals, viral stress may be enough to trigger FM.

In fact, research does suggest that a minority of people who develop viral diseases, which can include Lyme disease, Epstein-Barr (HHV-4), Herpes Lymphotropic Virus (HHV-6), Coxsackie B, Parvovirus, Hepatitis C, and HIV, may later go on to develop FM or CFIDS. Many people on the East Coast of the United States have been diagnosed with post-Lyme disease syndrome based on a positive blood test for Epstein-Barr. While the suffering of these patients is real, the diagnosis is now in question. Ongoing NIH-funded research suggests that many patients who have been treated at Lyme disease clinics may actually have FM, especially since multiple rounds of antibiotics and antiviral medication have failed to improve symptoms or physical functioning in these individuals. Regardless, the mechanism of how viruses may trigger FM in genetically higher-risk individuals merits further investigation.

Stress: Pathophysiological and Psychological Factors

Some patients report unrelenting stress as a precipitating factor in their development of FM. Stress in this case encompasses any kind of stressor, not just the response to emotional pain we typically may consider when we think of the term. Researchers now believe that stress can change human brain function. For example, studies in nonhuman primates have shown that exposure to psychosocial stressors results in changes to the tissues of the brain in the hippocampal complex. The hippocampus is a part of the forebrain, located in the medial temporal lobe, and belongs to the limbic system. The limbic system supports a variety of functions including emotion, behavior, and memory. People with hippocampal damage experience short-term memory problems and difficulty with spatial navigation, not unlike FM "fibro-fog" and FM balance issues. In fact, at least two studies using magnetic resonance spectroscopy have demonstrated metabolic abnormalities in the hippocampal complex in patients with FM that strongly correlate with their reported severity of clinical symptoms. Damage to the hippocampus does not affect other aspects of memory, such as the ability to learn new skills, which suggests that these other abilities depend on different brain regions than the hippocampus.

Autonomic Nervous System Dysfunction

The Autonomic Nervous System (ANS) is the portion of the nervous system that controls the function of organ systems for the body. Many think of it as the "automatic" nervous system because the mind does not rule its performance; it works below the conscious level. For instance, it regulates body temperature, blood pressure, breathing, heart rate, bowel and bladder tone, and myriad other functions necessary to maintain life. The peripheral autonomic system is divided into two branches: sympathetic and parasympathetic.

Sympathetic Nervous System

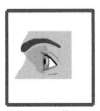

Dilates pupils

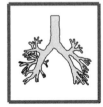

Relaxes airways

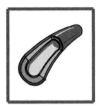

Constricts blood vessels

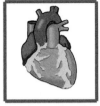

Accelerates heartbeat

Decreases salivation

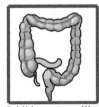

Inhibits gut motility and secretions

Stimulates secretion of epinephrine and norepinephrine

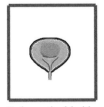

Relaxes the bladder

The goal of these two branches is to maintain equilibrium in many instances that range from life-threatening stress to deep sleep. Reactivity in the ANS is sometimes referred to as "fight or flight." The actions of the two branches of the ANS are determined by neurotransmitters (body chemicals originating in nerve cells and used to relay signals). Important neurotransmitters include adrenaline (also called norepinephrine, a stress hormone), which is the predominant

Parasympathetic Nervous System

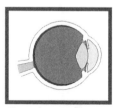

Constricts pupils

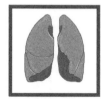

Constricts airways

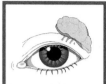

Stimulates secretion
from lachrymal gland

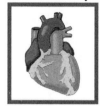

Slows heartbeat

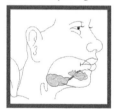

Stimulates salivation

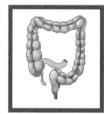

Stimulates gut motility

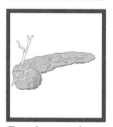

Exocrine secretions
stimulated

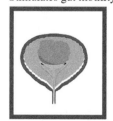

Stimulates urinary
bladder contraction

sympathetic neurotransmitter, and acetylcholine (another kind of stress hormone abbreviated as ACh), the main hormone responsible for regulating parasympathetic activity. Activity and reactions in the ANS can be measured by analyzing heart rate variability, which is often abnormal in people with FM. *Dysautonomia* is the medical term for ANS dysfunction, and there are medical researchers who believe it explains many, if not all, FM symptoms. This is because the hypothalamic-pituitary-adrenal axis, and specifically growth hormone, works closely with the ANS.

Precipitating Events and the Possible Role of Central Sensitization

Scientists know that a local injury resulting from trauma can lead to lingering pain. Pain that lasts for weeks, months, or years is termed *chronic pain* and is accompanied by changes in the chemical and anatomical makeup of the brain and spinal cord. Chronic pain that goes untreated can increase in intensity and spread from an original site to body areas that weren't previously affected, further damaging health and functioning. At that point, chronic pain becomes a disorder in itself. Why this happens in some people and not others is unclear, although genetics may play a role. What is certain is that sometimes an injury will lead to a constellation of changes, including an elevation of spontaneous CNS firing, an increase in pain response level and length, and a decrease of pain threshold. These are the changes collectively termed *central sensitization*, and they appear to be fundamental to the pain sensitivity that defines chronic pain.

To better understand central sensitization, knowledge of the functioning of the human nervous system is important. Neurons (nerve cells) are specific types of cells found only in the nervous system, and they contain receptors designed to send and receive signals. A neuron's receptors are the first to receive information regarding any harmful stimuli. This receptor information in turn travels the neural pathway from injury site to brain. When the information is transferred onward to those parts of the brain responsible for perception, the brain responds with pain signals that are returned to the most relevant body part, and at that point pain is felt in the location of origin. Pain receptors provide a simple response to an acute stimulus. This kind of simple pain is the everyday experience in response to injury, a signal to the body to move away from whatever may be causing injury. But these mechanisms responsible for simple pain do not explain pain that persists after healing has taken place or the source of pain is otherwise removed. Phantom limb pain is a good example of this kind of persistent pain response. The source of all possible sensation is obviously gone, but very real discomfort continues to be felt. Why does this happen?

The answer is that the nervous system includes both ascending excitatory and descending inhibitory neurotransmitters, and those two kinds of signals allow the body to react appropriately to both the start and the end of pain. When the inhibition phase of the nervous system response malfunctions, pain may continue to be felt. This takes place because neurons develop a "memory" of how to respond to the brain's electrical signals. The human body is advantageously set up in this way to respond rapidly and effectively when re-experiencing the same kinds of

Pain Processing Pathways

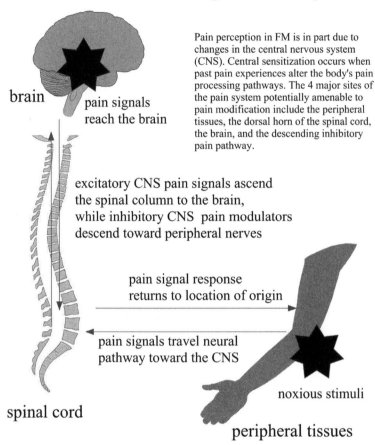

Pain perception in FM is in part due to changes in the central nervous system (CNS). Central sensitization occurs when past pain experiences alter the body's pain processing pathways. The 4 major sites of the pain system potentially amenable to pain modification include the peripheral tissues, the dorsal horn of the spinal cord, the brain, and the descending inhibitory pain pathway.

brain

pain signals
reach the brain

excitatory CNS pain signals ascend
the spinal column to the brain,
while inhibitory CNS pain modulators
descend toward peripheral nerves

pain signal response
returns to location of origin

pain signals travel neural
pathway toward the CNS

noxious stimuli

spinal cord

peripheral tissues

stimulation. Pain signals are an important part of this reaction, and while the nervous system's memory provides the protection of a quick response, it also can create abnormal reactions. Thus we see that when a person is injured, overstimulation of the neural receptors can produce a bigger and bigger response in the pain transmission pathways, and that pain causes further pain even as the stimulus that triggered the initial response has remained the same. Another problem in chronic pain is called the "expansion of receptive fields." This phenomenon occurs when previously undamaged tissue undergoes chemical and electrical changes that promote chronic pain. For example, if initially only the neck was painful, nearby areas like the shoulders may become involved as the "field of reception" is increased. In another example, researchers have found that newborns undergoing circumcision without anesthesia respond more profoundly to pain later in childhood. They exhibit a greater hemodynamic response (rapid heartbeat and breathing) to painful stimuli, such as routine injections, vaccinations, and other procedures. In the case of the chronic pain of fibromyalgia, it is the CNS inhibitory mechanisms that are thought to be faulty, so pain is both amplified inappropriately and is felt for an inordinate length of time. Other terms for this phenomenon are temporal summation and windup.

Lack of Restorative Sleep and the Possible Roles of Substance P and HPA Axis

In the 1990s, researchers proposed that exposure to stressful conditions could alter the function of the hypothalamic-pituitary-adrenal (HPA) axis, a major part of the neuroendocrine system that controls reactions to stress and regulates many body processes. Variations in HPA function are characterized by high levels of cortisol, which in turn is associated with the development of widespread pain. When cortisol excretion levels were measured in one research study, with a sample of forty-seven women diagnosed with FM compared to a control sample of fifty-eight healthy women of similar age, it was confirmed the women with FM excreted significantly lower cortisol levels than the healthy women. Other data in FM have demonstrated a blunted cortisol response to the stress of high-intensity exercise. Most recently, a lack of normal daily cortisol variation has been identified in FM.

Scientists theorize that Stage-4 sleep is critical to good nervous system function, because it is during that time the body releases needed neurochemicals. Deep sleep is thought to be critical in resetting levels of the neuropeptide Substance P, which is a key transmitter of pain to the brain. People with FM lack slow-wave sleep and often experience other factors that interfere with Stage-4 sleep such as pain, depression, anxiety, lack of serotonin, and RLS. According to the sleep disturbance hypothesis, a trauma or illness that causes sleep disturbance might trigger FM. Remember that chemical pain processing can be viewed as two opposing forces. The first process involves chemical messages sent to the brain that are interpreted as pain, and the second is a chemical response from the brain that attempts to inhibit the pain message. Pain sensations travel from the periphery to an area of the spinal cord called the dorsal horn, where the release of any chemicals, including Substance P, takes place. The chemicals released by the spinal cord work to attach themselves to neuroreceptors. Substance P binds itself to a receptor called NK1. The chemical message then travels upward along the spinal cord to the brain where the message is interpreted as pain. In response, the brain returns neurochemicals, such as serotonin, norepinephrine, zinc, and opioids, to the spinal cord where Substance P had been released. At this point there is a "down regulation" of Substance P that calms the perception of pain. Researchers believe that in FM this process is disrupted. A patient may have either too much Substance P or too few inhibitor chemicals. It is likely an imbalance of these chemicals plays an important part in the amplified pain cycle experienced in FM.

Another hypothesis suggests that reduced sleep leads to reduced production of human growth hormone (HGH) during slow-wave sleep. Many people with FM produce inadequate levels of HGH, and tests show that hormones under the direct or indirect control of HGH, including insulin-like growth factor 1 (IGF-1), cortisol, leptin, and neuropeptide Y are abnormal in people with FM. Most HGH is made during deep sleep, with additional pulsatile release throughout the day and in response to stress, such as vigorous exercise. Treatment with HGH has been shown to normalize IGF-1 and reduce symptoms in people with FM. Other medications have been demonstrated to improve HGH release in response to vigorous exercise but help only selected symptoms such as fatigue, sleep, anxiety, and ability to exercise. Research is ongoing regarding the best way to manipulate the HPA axis in order to return people with FM to better physical function.

Major Depressive Disorder

There is strong evidence that major depression is associated with FM, although the nature of the association has remained controversial. For example, some clinicians still hold that psychosomatic illness plays a large role in chronic pain conditions, including FM. In the past, clinicians endorsed a theory of Tension Myositis Syndrome (TMS). Practitioners who treat TMS consider that when pain cannot be relieved by standard medical treatments, psychosomatic illness is the likely cause, especially chronic pain in the back, neck, and limbs. The theory is that untreatable pain functions as an unconscious distraction from dangerous emotions, and when patients recognize this is the situation and confront their emotions, their symptoms no longer serve a useful purpose and go away. TMS treatment involves attitude change, education, and psychotherapy. Emerging objective evidence in pain processing in FM has led most researchers and clinicians away from TMS as an explanation for FM. Further, scientists are rejecting many of these psychologically-based theories of origin as they relate to FM.

In recent years, FM has been shown to have physical markers that rule out psychological illness as the lead cause of the disorder. Functional MRI imaging (fMRI) is a technique for visualizing metabolic activity in the brain in "real time." One study used fMRI to visualize brain responses to experimental pain among FM patients. It is important to note here that the sensation of pain has at least two sources: our sensory pathways process the magnitude of pain, whereas our affective pathways process the unpleasantness of pain. Depressive symptoms are associated with the magnitude of pain response in areas of the brain that specifically participate in affective pain processing but not in areas involved in sensory processing.

At least one of the FDA-indicated medications for FM has been demonstrated to work equally well in FM patients with or without depression. Since the FM subjects in the study showed pain response in the sensory processing portions of the brain, this is a good indication that the amplification of pain seen in FM is indeed independent of mood or emotion. While the majority of persons with FM do have a history of some depression, the incidence of psychiatric symptoms is still no higher than found in other chronic pain populations. In other words, there is no clear evidence that psychiatric illness causes FM. Further, while reviews of the relationship between FM and major depressive disorder (MDD) have found similarities between FM and MDD in neuroendocrine abnormalities, those findings do not support an assumption that MDD is the underlying disorder of FM.

Abnormal Neurotransmission: Serotonin, Norepinephrine, and Dopamine

Serotonin is a neurotransmitter that regulates sleep patterns, mood, a feeling of well-being, and inhibition of pain. Since those with FM experience abnormal pain, it has been hypothesized that the pathophysiology underlying FM may be an impairment of serotonin metabolism. This hypothesis is supported by finding decreased serotonin metabolites in FM patient plasma and cerebrospinal fluid. However, medications such as selective serotonin reuptake inhibitors (SSRIs, a type of antidepressant that acts on serotonin levels such as Zoloft and Prozac) do not seem to alleviate the majority of FM pain, whereas drugs such as mixed serotonin norepinephrine reuptake inhibitors (SNRIs, a type of antidepressant that acts on both serotonin and norepinephrine levels) seem to be more successful. Examples of SNRIs include the drugs Cymbalta (duloxetine) and Savella (milnacipran) that also have been used to treat depression and the pain of diabetic neuropathy with some success.

Central Dopamine Dysfunction: COMT Gene Disruption

Dopamine plays a critical role in pain perception and pain relief. It is a catecholamine neurotransmitter perhaps best known for its various roles in Parkinson's disease, schizophrenia, and drug addiction. It also appears related to Restless Legs Syndrome (RLS), which is a common co-morbidity in patients with FM. The theory of central dopamine dysfunction suggests that the main abnormality responsible for FM symptoms is disrupted dopamine neurotransmission. This conclusion supposes that FM is characterized by low levels of central dopamine resulting from both genetic factors and an exposure to environmental stressors. These stressors might include physical trauma, viral infections, inflammatory disorders like rheumatoid arthritis and SLE, or psychosocial distress. There are three points of reasoning to this theory: first, chronic exposure to stress results in a disruption of dopamine-related neurotransmission; second, FM patients fail to release adequate dopamine in response to pain; third, a number of FM patients in drug research studies have responded well to dopamine agonists, such as Pramipexole, which is currently used to treat Parkinson's disease and Restless Legs Syndrome.

In conclusion, exciting new research into FM is under way. The multiple objective abnormalities identified and reproduced in FM over the past three decades spur scientists on in their quest to better understand this disorder. And it is most fortunate that previous research has shown FM can no longer be labeled merely a psychosomatic disorder. Remaining skeptics point to a lack of a single hypothetical framework as their rationale for not believing that FM is real. The next critical challenge is for researchers to combine all of the earlier-mentioned abnormal findings into a testable model that will explain the totality of FM.

4

Treatment by Health Providers

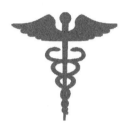

By definition, no single surgery or round of medications will cure a chronic illness. Since that is the case, treatments for chronic illnesses are ongoing and lifelong. A bio-psycho-social treatment schedule has proved to be the best approach for regaining good quality of life when living with FM.

The ultimate goal of health treatment is to reduce symptoms, promote physical fitness, and optimize the ability to perform activities of daily living. One health-care provider alone cannot hope to accomplish this breadth of goals. An interdisciplinary team of providers is generally required for the best treatment outcome. The most important player on the team, however, is the person with FM. A patient who is active in the management of his or her FM is critical. A passive person with FM who expects a doctor will cure them will be disappointed. The FM patient who is proactive in his or her own health will need to assemble a treatment team and, further, become well educated about their own disorder. This will mean staying informed about any current medication and its possible side effects, learning about common FM co-morbidity symptoms, exploring cognitive behavioral strategies along with complementary and alternative therapies, participating in exercise, and maintaining a nutritional diet. A good treatment team can provide the necessary knowledge.

ASSEMBLING A TREATMENT TEAM

The Primary Provider

A single primary provider who can prescribe medications is the cornerstone of the treatment team. This might be a nurse practitioner, physician's assistant, family practice physician, internist, osteopathic physician (a holistic provider also called a doctor of osteopathy, or DO), or perhaps a physiatrist (a physician specializing in physical rehabilitation). The primary provider will be responsible for making the diagnosis, prescribing medications, and managing recommendations from other specialists. Other key members of the team include a physical therapist (PT), an occupational therapist (OT), a speech therapist (ST), a clinical exercise specialist (CES), a psychologist, and a registered dietitian (RD). Optimally, they are employed by the same institution or health-care practice and can then work together efficiently on evaluation, treatment, and ongoing care. Their skill sets are both complementary and overlapping. One way PT, OT, ST, CES, and RD team members might divide treatment and care is as follows:

The Physical Therapist (PT)

A PT can evaluate and treat regional pain, balance issues, and discuss energy conservation to manage fatigue. Treatments employed by PTs may include rehabilitation exercise, manual therapies, neurosensory balance analyses (measuring nerve transmission information to and from peripheral extremities to the CNS), gait analyses with corrective orthotics fitting, and a multitude of management strategies for long-term self-care. They can also teach patients to use spray-and-stretch. Spray-and-stretch requires a prescription from the provider for fluoromethasone cooling spray (a skin refrigerant). The PT can teach patients to spray the medication on selected muscles, which allows painfully tight muscles to be stretched with less discomfort. Patients can then use spray-and-stretch at home whenever needed. PTs may fit patients for prescription orthotics for foot pain and work in concert with an orthotist to ensure proper fitting. Finally, PTs may administer ultrasound therapies to reduce pain from regional syndromes, including temporomandibular joint dysfunction (also called TMD, a cause of jaw pain) and chronic back pain.

The Occupational Therapist (OT)

An OT can provide many of the same services as a physical therapist but commonly will focus more on physical modifications to workplace, home, or activities of daily living. Some PTs/OTs will divide the care of FM patients so that large muscle/joints are evaluated and managed by the PT while smaller muscles/joints are evaluated by the OT. An example of this could include management of wrist pain or carpal tunnel by the OT and management of knee pain by the PT. In addition to providing individually fitted wrist splints and rehabilitative exercises, the OT might train the patient in such things as how to keep the body aligned in a neutral position during normal activity. The OT also has ergonomic expertise and can recommend a variety of equipment to ease pain and promote optimal posture. The OT is usually well versed in creating an optimal work environment. They can help patients ask employers for special accommodations such as avoidance of bright or flashing lights, strong smells, cold environments, or loud noises. They can help clarify whether an employee can physically tolerate standing for prolonged periods of time, can perform repetitive tasks, and has a fast, unobstructed path to the restroom, and they can explain the need for that employee to take short, frequent stretch breaks. At home, they can help patients think twice about where they store commonly used items in the kitchen, how to hang pictures, and how to do housework, and they can remind their patient of the need to pace themselves to avoid triggering a symptom flare. They are often the providers who suggest modifications such as vocational rehabilitation or suggest that patients consider disability.

The Speech Therapist (ST)

The ST is a communications expert who can also evaluate cognitive difficulties such as "fibro-fog" and differentiate them from cognitive deficits related to dementia, post-stroke, or head trauma. FM patients often report great distress about their perceived cognitive decline, so the ability to improve cognitive function is typically welcomed as life-enhancing. The ST will recommend a variety of nonpharmacologic strategies to maximize cognitive abilities and provide mental exercises to help enhance memory. Some of these strategies include establishing easily recalled routines, placing reminder notes, forming memory associations, decreasing multitasking, and reducing distractions.

The Clinical Exercise Specialist (CES)

The CES is a fitness professional who has advanced training in working with special populations, including those with chronic illnesses. In this developing field, the CES works as a bridge between the medical clinic and a home or public exercise setting where ongoing postrehabilitative workouts can take place. They provide guidance that takes into account the recommendations of the primary provider, the PT, the OT, and the ST. The CES may work as a specialized in-home personal trainer or lead special population classes in a general exercise setting. They also work as medical research study team members, providing physical function testing or leading strictly defined study-based group exercise. In their close association with an FM client, they are often the first to hear about side effects or adverse events that might be related to a prescription drug, a developing co-morbidity, or a change in disease course. They are an important link in knowledge and communication, encouraging a client with FM to seek direction and further treatment planning from the primary provider or other members of the treatment team.

The Psychologist

The psychologist is one of many health-care providers who can help maximize quality of life in someone with a chronic illness. Similarly, psychiatric mental health nurse practitioners (PMHNPs) and medical social workers (MSWs) possess some of the same skill set. All can generally offer counseling related to cognitive behavioral strategies. These strategies are often beyond the scope of the primary health-care provider. Cognitive behavioral strategies are formed by "talk therapy" and are individualized for each patient. For many with FM, these therapies can include fatigue control, decreasing catastrophic thinking, and boundary setting. There are numerous other types of counseling as well that these professionals can employ, depending on the needs of the patient or family they are treating. The PMHNP can also prescribe medication to augment therapy.

The Registered Dietitian (RD)

The RD is helpful in FM because many people's quality of life will improve through dietary change. The RD can help people learn not only what foods to avoid or minimize but how to introduce new foods into the diet and how to really enjoy those new foods. In FM, obesity is often a problem, especially due to the sporadic nature of FM flare cycles and the resulting disruption of an exercise routine. The RD can individualize an eating plan based on each patient's food preferences. In general, they discourage "diets" and emphasize healthier eating for the long run. They also try to strip away moral value from food by discouraging naming certain foods "good" or "bad." Instead, they focus on which foods to eat often and which foods to enjoy less frequently or in smaller amounts. Another role of the RD is to help people with concurrent celiac disease since gluten and its related products are so prevalent in the food supply. Lactose intolerance is a bit easier to negotiate, but an RD will have tips to minimize symptoms stemming from that problem as well. The future of RDs in FM can involve helping patients remove or reduce dietary excitotoxins, including agents such as unbound glutamate. Similarly, as evidence mounts regarding agents such as aspartame and its influence on NDMA receptor activity, those foods may need to be modified as well. These last two are particularly tricky because dietary excitotoxins are common in our food supply but are not generally listed on food labels. When they are listed, they come in a variety of names and chemical compounds. The term *nutritionist* is not protected by law; therefore, anyone can claim the title of nutritionist, including many diet authors. The title of RD or LD (registered and licensed dietitians) guarantees qualification by license and legal standards. Unfortunately, many third-party payers (insurance companies) do not reimburse RDs for working with patients who have a chronic illness. Reimbursement payments are often limited to diabetics and those with end-stage renal disease. FM patients can persist or they can set aside pretax dollars in employee-sponsored flexible health care spending accounts, thereby reducing the tax burden of spending out of pocket on a chronic illness.

The Co-Morbidity Specialists

Others who can bring optimal care are the medical providers who specialize in the common co-morbidities of FM. It is critical for the primary provider to seek evaluation and treatment recommendations for any diagnosed or undiagnosed symptom within the specialist's area of expertise. The primary provider does not ask the specialist to manage the patient's overall FM; he or she only refers the patient for treatment of the co-morbidity.

The Gastroenterologist

One specialist that may be called on is a gastroenterologist (a specialist in the digestive system and its disorders), also commonly known as a "GI doctor." A gastroenterologist may be helpful for people with GI distress such as irritable bowel syndrome that does not respond to traditional therapies. Ideally, the gastroenterologist would screen for other GI conditions such as inflammatory bowel disease or celiac disease (autoimmune disorders that are often genetic), symptomatic diverticulitis (inflamed areas in the intestinal lining), and peptic ulcer disease (caused by erosions to the lining of the digestive system). Many patients who are diagnosed by a gastroenterologist with irritable bowel syndrome find it reassuring that their GI distress is not caused by a malignancy like cancer or any other progressive illness.

The Urologist

A urologist (a specialist focusing on the urinary tracts of men and women and on the reproductive system of men) may be helpful for patients with severe irritable bladder. Like other specialists, they can rule out malignant and progressive diseases and reassure the patient that irritable bladder is the correct diagnosis. Many times specialists are aware of therapies that are not FDA-indicated for the treatment of various ailments. For example, some patients find some degree of relief from irritable bladder with a combination of prescription medications used concurrently with suprapubic transcutaneous nerve stimulation (a transcutaneous electrical nerve stimulator, commonly called a TENS unit, which is used to apply electrical current through the skin for pain control). A gynecologist or urogynecologist may also have expertise in managing pelvic pain syndromes such as endometriosis, severe dysmenorrhea (painful menstruation), vulvodynia (burning, stinging, or irritation of the female genitalia), and vulvar vestibulitis (redness and pain in a specific region of the female genitalia). Men may also suffer from frequent or painful urination or a painful prostate (prostadynia). These conditions severely impact not only the patient's quality of life but spill over into their sexual relationships. Long-term partner relationships for persons with FM have sometimes dissolved due to gynecologic co-morbidities. Moreover, lack of libido is not uncommon in FM. Gynecologists are also expert in hormone perimenopausal or postmenopausal hormone replacement. Until recently, primary-care providers routinely prescribed estrogen with or without progesterone to reduce menopause symptoms and promote bone and blood vessel health. A large-scale study has now cast doubt on the wisdom of prescribing hormone therapy for all women. As specialists in their field, gynecologists can better prescribe these medications selectively, depending on patients' symptoms and risk factors.

The Sleep Medicine Physician

Physicians who have studied in this subspecialty can administer and interpret a sleep study. Sleep studies are critical for patients with signs or symptoms suggestive of sleep apnea (a disorder characterized by pauses and gasps while breathing during sleep) or narcolepsy (a neurological condition characterized by extreme tiredness and/or falling asleep during the day at inappropriate times). Symptoms of sleep deprivation may include extreme daytime sleepiness, going to sleep while driving, loud snoring with pauses between breaths, and waking with an occipital headache (pain in the back of the skull and radiating down the neck). Sleep medicine physicians may or may not be interested in treating chronic insomnia. Some are comfortable with providing a long-term prescription of controlled substance sleep agents; others will rely instead on sleep hygiene, tricyclic or SSRI medications, and referral for cognitive behavioral therapy.

The Endocrinologist

An endocrinologist might be called on if a patient with FM has any of the following four conditions: 1) thyroid dysfunction not controlled with standard therapies, 2) peripheral neuropathy, 3) hormone deficiencies such as low HGH and testosterone, and 4) statin intolerance due to musculoskeletal pain. Some endocrinologists have expertise regarding human growth hormone (HGH) deficiency in adults. Those who are interested in treating HGH will most likely order a growth hormone stimulation test. The most common HGH test involves delivering an acute dose of growth-hormone-releasing hormone and arginine (a common natural amino acid). Growth hormone is released by the pituitary gland in response to the drug challenge, and then measured in the blood three to five times over several hours. If the patient fails to produce adequate HGH, they may be diagnosed with adult growth hormone deficiency syndrome and thus be eligible for third-party reimbursement for daily growth hormone injections. Growth hormone is produced with expensive recombinant DNA technology, and the price can be prohibitive unless insurance offsets part of the cost. This form of treatment is generally lifelong. Another hormone replacement that is sometimes used in FM is testosterone. Many older men on chronic opioid analgesics (strong pain relief medications) have low levels of testosterone in their blood and experience fatigue and muscular deconditioning. Endocrinologists can often help patients weigh the risks versus benefits of testosterone replacement therapy. Statin intolerance occurs when a patient with hyperlipidemia (raised or abnormal levels of lipids such as cholesterol or triglycerides in the bloodstream) cannot tolerate the drugs used to reduce LDL levels, which in turn help control cardiovascular diseases. Specialists who prescribe a wide variety of statin- and other blood-lipid-lowering medications may know which statins are least likely to contribute to muscle pain, or may be able to prescribe very low-dose statins in combination with other lipid-lowering agents that will serve to bypass the side effect of muscle pain. It is critical that patients with FM not be allowed to develop vascular disease due to lack of treatment. The consequences of untreated hyperlipidemia may include highly invasive cardiac bypass surgery, stroke, or pain in the extremities caused by PAD (peripheral artery disease).

The Neurologist

A neurologist may be called to rule out other conditions that worry patients. For example, many young women with FM become concerned they actually have multiple sclerosis (MS). A neurologist is adroit at identifying this kind of neurodegenerative disease. The more common problem encountered by people with FM that is treatable by a neurologist is chronic headache. Many neurologists have extensive experience diagnosing and managing a variety of headaches. Decreasing the frequency and severity of headaches may not only improve the patient's quality of life but may in turn help reduce the central pain of fibromyalgia. Some argue that because the brain, spinal cord, and peripheral nerves are adversely affected in FM, neurologists should be the primary providers for people with FM. In reality, there are currently too few neurologists to accept the additional patient load. Primary care is therefore argued to be the best home for fibromyalgia, with continued referral to neurologists to rule out other problems.

The Rheumatologist

The rheumatologist is a specialist who manages autoimmune rheumatic diseases, such as rheumatoid arthritis (an autoimmune disease causing joint pain and deformity), and degenerative joint diseases such as osteoarthritis (an inflammation that causes joint pain). It is common for patients with FM to have stiff joints that feel swollen, but they should not have inflammation, synovitis (fluid around the joints), or signs of major joint degeneration. FM patients who see rheumatologists may be given a blood test called the antinuclear antibody test (ANA) that diagnoses systemic lupus erythematosus (SLE, a chronic, inflammatory autoimmune disorder affecting any one of the following: skin, joints, blood cells, kidneys, heart, lungs). There is a high false-positive rate for this test, which is a source of great stress for many FM patients who inaccurately assume that they have SLE. For this reason, ANA testing is best reserved for patients whose history and physical exam does specifically suggest SLE. Conversely, it is interesting how many people at first say they would prefer to have a diagnosis of SLE over FM. This preference changes rapidly when they learn the former is potentially life-threatening. FM may coexist with other rheumatic conditions such as rheumatoid arthritis, systemic lupus, and Sjögren's Syndrome, but the treatments for these autoimmune conditions are different than treatments for FM. Osteoarthritis of the knee and hip may be treated with injections and local therapies. The rheumatologist will also know when it is appropriate to refer the patient to an orthopedic surgeon for evaluation for joint replacement.

The Orthopedic Surgeon

Orthopedic surgeons are experts at evaluating joints and bones and determining if a surgical intervention would be helpful. Every person with FM has spine pain since it is part of the diagnostic criteria, but FM patients are referred for spine evaluation by the primary provider when neurologic signs and *severe* symptoms are evident. Spinal surgery is successful in the right patient, for the right diagnosis, such as spinal stenosis (abnormal narrowing). However, outcomes for spinal surgery designed to eliminate pain, when done in the absence of neurological signs, may be disappointing to the patient. For instance, neurosurgeons are sometimes asked to evaluate persons with FM for Chiari (pronounced kee-AR-ee) malformation. Chiari malformation is an anatomical problem in which part of the brainstem protrudes downward toward the spinal column. Research has shown that only a small number of patients with FM have anatomic abnormalities consistent with a Chiari malformation confirmed by clinical signs. Research also has demonstrated a lack of correlation between clinical examinations and MRI findings of Chiari malformation. Therefore, neurosurgery for most people with FM is typically not helpful.

The Psychiatrist

A psychiatrist or other mental health provider such as a psychiatric mental health nurse practitioner (PMHNP), medical social worker, or psychologist can be helpful with co-morbid mood disorders that do not respond to the standard therapies used in primary care. Unipolar disorder (depression without mood swings), anxiety disorder, and posttraumatic stress disorder (PTSD, an anxiety disorder that develops after exposure to an ordeal) are more common in FM than the general population. There is additional evidence that a mild form of bipolar disorder (mood swings that move from depression to exaggerated happiness) may also be overrepresented in FM. Any of the psychiatric providers mentioned earlier can diagnose these conditions and provide cognitive behavioral therapies and other counseling strategies to improve symptoms. Additionally, a psychiatrist or PMHNP can prescribe medications for mood disorders. Because sleep disorders such as insomnia are common in mental health conditions, these providers are also excellent long-term prescribers of sleep medications. Lastly, persons with Axis II disorders (personality disorders and ailments such as schizophrenia) should be managed by a psychiatrist. To date, Axis II disorders are not thought to be overrepresented in FM. Conversely, people with these diagnoses might develop FM and so require co-morbid psychiatric management.

PATIENT EDUCATION

After assembling the FM treatment team, education about FM is invaluable. Education can occur individually between the provider and patient, in support groups, or through carefully selected books, media, and Internet sites. The primary provider is tasked with providing education regarding the validity of the FM diagnosis and the nondestructive nature of the condition on muscle. The provider outlines a rational treatment plan focusing on minimizing symptoms and restoring functionality. It is disheartening to learn that it is generally not possible to return to the state of health experienced before the onset of FM; most symptoms can never be totally eradicated. Having realistic expectations about the amount of relief possible from medications (generally 30 to 50 percent) is important for learning to cope with a new lifestyle reality. The primary provider will be supportive but realistic in terms of the life-long nature of FM. Together patient and provider can review evidence-based educational materials. Touted "cures" can be discussed between the primary provider and the patient, but ultimately treatment choices and financial decisions belong to the patient.

Armed with a treatment team and knowledge about the disorder, the patient can begin to make lifestyle modifications. For severely affected persons, this may mean reducing the hours of work done inside and outside the home. Patients with invisible chronic illnesses, including FM, often get little support because they do not look sick. Patients often feel guilty about how FM has limited their lives and how it affects their family and friendships. To manage their disorder, they must learn to be more assertive in declining extra tasks and invitations. For example, a holiday tradition that includes eight extra family members visiting as house guests may need to be changed; a better plan may be meeting daily for a few hours at a restaurant or other location outside the home over two to four days. In well-managed FM, fatigue control becomes an important strategy. This means on occasion limiting chores to those that are most essential or deciding on just one of several possible fun activities. Energy-saving techniques can include simple changes such as sitting during showering or while brushing teeth. Many with FM have great difficulty with activities that require them to hold their arms at shoulder height or higher for long periods. Therefore, a woman with FM might need to opt for a hairstyle that doesn't require a great deal of hair drying and styling.

In summary, assembling the health-care team is the key to optimizing outcomes in FM. The primary provider will shoulder the burden of medication adjustments and provide rational and timely referrals. The other key treatment team members are assembled as additional advisors for optimal daily living, while the specialist team takes care of co-morbidity challenges. But the most important person for a successful life is the patient, who becomes the well-informed advocate for his or her own health.

5

Pharmacological and Nonpharmacological Treatments

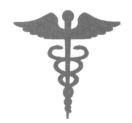

MEDICATIONS FOR FM

At the time of this writing, more than 100 clinical trials have been conducted testing various medications for the treatment of FM. A few of those medications have been indicated for FM. A drug is termed *indicated* when the Food and Drug Administration (FDA) formally announces that research has shown a certain drug to be helpful for a specific condition. Central sensitization contributes to an enhancement of side effects from medication. Because of this, people with FM are directed to "start low and go slow" when starting any new medications. In other words, if the usual recommended dose of medication is 60 mg per day, the person with FM may need to begin their treatment at 20 mg for a week, increase to 30 mg for the next week, and then finally move to the target dose of 60 mg on the third week. Many people with FM have suspected at one time or another they have multiple drug allergies, but in reality almost all of these reactions are proven to be CNS-enhanced side effects (e.g., nausea, vomiting, dizziness), rather than life-threatening anaphylactic (allergic) reactions. The broad categories of prescription medications for FM include: 1) pain medications, 2) mood medications, and 3) sleep medications.

Pain Medications

The simplest form of pain medications includes over-the-counter acetaminophen (*ah-seat-ah-MIN-oh-fen*), ibuprofen (*eye-bee-PRO-fen*), and aspirin. These might come marketed in solo form or in a combination, and with or without the addition of caffeine. Nearly all people with FM take these medications due to their accessibility and low cost. Unfortunately, their efficacy in clinical trials has been shown to be minimal.

The Drug Enforcement Administration (DEA) is a U.S. government watchdog agency. One of this agency's major tasks is to restrict potentially harmful prescription drug availability to U.S. citizens. The DEA has established a controlled-substance system with rankings called "schedules," which lists both legal and illegal drugs. For legal drugs, scheduling serves to keep potentially dangerous prescription medication distribution in check. Controlled substances can range from Schedule I (the most addictive, such as LSD and heroin) to Schedule V (the least addictive, including medications such as pregabalin and certain cough syrups).

The first FDA-indicated medication for FM was pregabalin (*pre-GAB-ahl-in*), which is an anticonvulsant. Anticonvulsant medications that are classified as CNS depressants also can be useful in treating pain. Side effects to pregabalin include drowsiness, lightheadedness, and potential weight gain; however, initially feeling sleepy or dizzy when first starting this medication typically goes away after a certain period of continuing on the medication. Taking a higher dose at bedtime and a lower dose in the morning can also minimize these undesirable side effects.

Opioid (*OH-pea-oyd*) medications are generally used for severe pain. Natural opiates include morphine and codeine. Some of the more commonly known synthetic opioids are heroin, fentanyl (*FEN-tan-ill*), and hydrocodone (*hi-drow-CO-dohn*). These medications are commonly used to treat FM but are limited by side effects such as nausea, vomiting, constipation, and worsening of fibro-fog. A further serious complication of opiate treatment includes what is termed *dose escalation and tolerance*. This means that over time a patient will need to take higher and higher doses for the same amount of relief. An even further, albeit rare, complication of dose escalation and tolerance is opioid-induced hyperalgesia (increased sensitivity to pain). This is a situation in which increased doses of opiates actually begin to worsen pain.

Mood Medications

Antidepressant medications (commonly referred to as mood medications) can take many forms. Some only improve depression and anxiety, whereas others improve pain and promote sleep as well as mood. Three major classes of mood medications are used in the treatment of FM: tricyclic antidepressants, SSRIs, and SNRIs.

In the 1970s and 1980s, tricyclic antidepressants such as Elavil (*EL-eh-vill*) were commonly used in FM. Unfortunately, tricyclic antidepressants are associated with side effects such as dry eyes, dry mouth, constipation, weight gain, daytime sleepiness, and dose escalation and tolerance. Patients who were willing to accept those side effects did experience moderate improvement for multiple symptoms. However, with the advent of newer antidepressant medications, tricyclics are used less often today. One exception is low-dose tricyclics that are commonly prescribed at bedtime for people with very mild FM.

The next class of mood medication was introduced in the 1990s. The selective serotonin reuptake inhibitors (SSRIs) in the earliest form helped mood and sleep but gave minimal improvement in pain. Prozac was the first drug in this class. Each successive SSRI coming to the market provided enhancements, becoming more selective for serotonin reuptake. Still, drugs in this class only improve mood and are therefore not widely recommended for the treatment of pain in FM.

The contemporary management of FM has seen a switch from prescribing SSRIs to a newer class of mood medication called selective serotonin and norepinephrine reuptake inhibitors (SNRIs). This class of drug treats the pain and fatigue of FM independent of its effect on improving mood and is proving a better fit for the majority of FM patients. Duloxetine (*Duh-LOCKS-eh-teen*) is an SNRI, and in 2008 it became the second FDA-indicated drug for the treatment of FM. Milnaciprin is the newest SNRI to have received FDA approval for fibromyalgia. Even newer drugs that only reuptake norepinephrine are currently under study in research drug trials.

Sleep Medications

In 1975, a Canadian sleep researcher demonstrated that he could induce FM-like symptoms in healthy college students by startling them into wakefulness with a 90dB siren during Stage-4 sleep, also commonly termed the *alpha-delta sleep state*. In these healthy subjects, Stage-4 sleep deprivations caused musculoskeletal and mood symptoms comparable to the symptoms seen in FM, and symptoms stopped after allowing the students to return to their normal, restorative sleep patterns. Since that research result, treating sleep has been crucial to managing FM. However, medications best for sleep are controlled substances, and some primary providers are hesitant to prescribe controlled substances long-term.

Drugs to promote sleep include short-acting hypnotics such as benzodiazepines (*ben-zoh-die-AZ-eh-peens*) and, most recently, a medication that increases time in the alpha-delta sleep state called Xyrem (*ZIE-rehm*). Xyrem is currently FDA-indicated for hypersomnia (excessive daytime sleepiness or prolonged nighttime sleep) associated with the cataplexy (seizure symptoms) that comes with narcolepsy (falling asleep at inappropriate times). In FM clinical trials to date, Xyrem appears to normalize sleep and thereby improves multiple FM symptoms including pain and fatigue.

Other Medications Used in FM

Muscle relaxants are often prescribed in FM due to complaints of muscle stiffness, spasm, and pain. They are minimally effective but commonly employed nonetheless. One drug with muscle-relaxing qualities called tinzanidine (*tin-ZAN-eh-deen*) performed well in clinical trials but requires ongoing monitoring of liver enzymes during its use.

Cyclobenzaprine (*sigh-clo-BEN-zah-preen*) is often thought to be a muscle relaxant, but chemically it is more aligned with tricyclic antidepressants. Used at night, cyclobenzaprine may help people with mildly disordered sleep. Unfortunately, when used during the day, it can contribute to fatigue or fibro-fog. Dopamine agonists (compounds that mimic the effect of the neurotransmitter dopamine) are increasingly used in FM. At low doses they are helpful for Restless Legs Syndrome (RLS). At higher doses they can treat many of the symptoms of FM. Stimulants such as Ritalin that are commonly used in attention deficit disorder (ADD) are sometimes prescribed for daytime fatigue and fibro-fog, though currently there is scant evidence to support the use of these agents.

In Appendix A, a list of alphabetized commonly used medications in FM is presented with brand and generic names, dose ranges, clinical prescribing pearls, and a real-life story about a patient taking each prescribed item.

NONPHARMACOLOGICAL TREATMENTS

Although standard Western medicine's pharmacological treatments for FM are a common starting point to reclaiming a sense of control over this disorder, there are many more tools available that can serve to improve quality of life. Since chronic illness is almost always lifelong, looking for additional coping strategies is a quite realistic approach.

Cognitive Behavioral Strategies

Cognitive behavioral strategies are a skill set used to minimize symptom severity and reduce unhelpful thinking. Many people, when first diagnosed with FM, experience an existential crisis that may last several years. This crisis has to do with loss of their previous "selves" and acceptance of their new "selves." The cognitive/behavioral strategies outlined on the following pages work to help the newly diagnosed move toward acceptance of their changed lifestyle and can ultimately improve their quality of life. The first strategy is pacing.

In U.S. society most activities are based on task completion rather than time allocation. For example, if a person needs to paint a wall or write a report for work, they typically will continue toiling at this task until it is completed. An alternative way to accomplish an activity is called "timed-based" pacing. It is quite useful when physical fatigue is a factor that must be reckoned with. Every twenty to thirty minutes during the day, people with FM are told to stop their current task and either rest or move their body in a different fashion. Rest would be appropriate if the task is physical; movement would be appropriate if the task is sedentary (e.g., working at the computer). Because of our societal expectations, this skill is difficult for many persons to master and may at first require people to use watch alarms or other cueing devices that will remind them to take a scheduled break. Understandably, time-based pacing can seem fragmented and frustrating. People generally want to finish a task, but in FM such behavior can easily result in a symptom flare. The key to acceptance of time-based pacing as a work strategy occurs when those with FM realize that by avoiding debilitating flares, they will actually accomplish more in the long run.

Another cognitive behavioral strategy is the scheduling of pleasant activities. This may sound silly to someone without a chronic illness, but people with FM often find their lives becoming smaller and their pool of friends and support people shrinking. People with FM often cannot tolerate long days of physical activity such as a full-day hike or lengthy travel. Even seemingly nonphysically challenging events like meeting friends for dinner may prove impossible if every bit of energy reserve is gone by the end of the day. There are two important components in successfully scheduling pleasant activities. The first is to develop a pool of activities that are realistic. This may mean finding new hobbies. Perhaps running needs to be replaced with walking; extensive on-the-go travel needs be changed to go-and-rest trips that allow more downtime; gardening a large plot may need to be replaced with other nature enjoyments such as bird-watching or photography.

Understandably, people with FM are concerned about what the future holds for them. Quite a few people with FM enjoyed healthy childhoods and young adulthoods. They are often well educated and involved with careers, their community, and raising families. When FM suddenly hits, they are generally helpless in their attempts to return to life before FM, and they often wonder, "How could everything go so wrong so quickly"? In cases of sudden FM onset, a determined effort is often required to steer clear of catastrophic thinking. Catastrophic thinking occurs when people begin to worry about outcomes that are unlikely or otherwise out of proportion to the problem at hand. For example, people with FM may worry that they will lose everything: their jobs, their homes, their families, their friends, and their lives. This scenario is exceedingly unlikely. The goal in cognitive therapy for removing catastrophic thinking is to recognize it and replace it with more realistic thoughts. People can ask themselves: "How likely is this problem to occur?" "What is the worst thing that can happen if it does occur?" "What is more likely to happen if this problem occurs?" and "What small steps can I take to reduce the likelihood that this problem will occur?" Because catastrophic thinking can gradually become second nature, people may have to revisit this coping skill over time and continue to practice replacing less helpful thought patterns with more realistic and optimistic ones.

Another cognitive behavioral skill set involves sleep hygiene. Sleep hygiene refers to all nonpharmacologic activities that people can do to maximize sleep efficiency. For people who have never had difficulty falling asleep or staying asleep, the concept of sleep hygiene might seem odd and unnecessary; after all, don't people just close their eyes and go to sleep? Sleep hygiene becomes necessary when physiologic processes degrade sleep. Techniques to enhance sleep include the following:

- remove pets from the bedroom;
- move to a new sleep location if a bed partner snores;
- use silicone ear plugs;
- install blackout curtains;
- go to bed at a regular time each night;
- routinely take a warm bath one hour before bedtime;
- keep computers and other work-related activities out of the bedroom;
- rest or nap in a different location to reserve the bed for sleeping;
- avoid stimulating activities such as TV news, bill paying, or arguing near bedtime; and
- do gentle stretching and deep breathing exercises near bedtime

Exercise

The FM patient who has difficulty walking to the mailbox and back without fatigue may have a hard time believing that an exercise program will ever become something to look forward to, or further, might someday provide relief from their pain. However once pain levels are made stable by medications to restore sleep and reduce pain, an exercise program needs to be started. The reasons include the following four points: first, people with chronic pain who exercise regularly often require less pain medication for the same amount of pain relief; second, specific exercises can brace and ease sore joints by taking the load off bones and cartilage; third, stronger muscles are less prone to muscle micro trauma which also will lessen daily pain; finally, exercise done on a regular basis improves sleep and will provide more energy over the long-term for those with chronic pain. The importance of exercise is not limited to its ability to increase flexibility, strength, and endurance. Inactivity brings on a cycle of deconditioning that can prove debilitating. The FM patient who tries to "hold still so it won't hurt" is actually allowing muscles to atrophy (wither through disuse). As muscles and joints weaken, and as the heart and lungs become unused to working under stress, ever-decreasing levels of physical ability are the result. In other words, the patient who started out trying to hold still to avoid pain eventually feels pain even when holding still.

There are special exercising techniques that will minimize postexercise pain in FM. A slow progression is needed, along with an avoidance of excessive eccentric muscle work (working the muscle while it lengthens). For this reason, downhill sports can prove unusually difficult because certain leg muscles are placed in an eccentric pattern when moving downward. Similarly, exercises such as advanced yoga and activities such as skiing that force the FM participant to hold one challenging position for long lengths of time could cause muscle fatigue that does not go away for days. Repetitive movements are also problematic because of the muscle challenge they present. A workout that frequently alters exercise patterns will help avoid the resulting postexertional muscle pain.

An exercise program that is ideal for FM might begin with relearning breathing patterns. Individuals with chronic pain often unconsciously hold their bodies in a tight position, which can result in shallow breathing. This disordered breathing in turn promotes a loss of the ability to relax even when pain abates. The next phase of exercise incorporates restoring good postural alignment. Typical pain postures include shoulders high held toward the ears and forward of the anatomical position. This misalignment of the shoulders can increase neck tension, as well as keeping the pectoral (chest) muscles short and tight and, conversely, keeping the upper back muscles, the so-called "posture muscles," stretched and unsupportive. Persons who are in pain tend to do a great deal of sitting. Over time the hip flexors, powerful muscles in the front of the torso that connect the torso to the hips, can shorten with prolonged sitting. At the same time, the muscles in the back of the thighs will become tight and contribute to poor alignment. These changes can be accompanied by weak abdominal and erector spinae (the muscles that run near the spinal column) muscles, a leading contributor to low back pain.

Correcting postural imbalance takes both flexibility work for the body's tight muscles and strength training to improve tone in the weakened muscles. Muscles to stretch for postural benefits include: the pectoral (chest), the anterior deltoids (front of the shoulders), the hip flexors and quadriceps (torso-to-hip connectors and front of the thighs), the gluteus medius (backside muscles that sit near the sciatic nerve), the hamstrings (back of the thighs), and the gastrocnemius and soleus (calf muscles). Muscles to strengthen include: the trapezius (upper back), posterior deltoids (back of the shoulders), rhomboids (between the shoulder blades), latissimus dorsi (mid back), erector spinae and abdominals (back and front of the lower torso and pelvic girdle), and the tibialis anterior muscle (front of the lower leg).

When breathing and posture are functioning well, balance training can be of great help for FM. Typical balance work includes one-legged stances and, later, the addition of soft surfaces, such as spongy balance pads, to provide further challenge. This training has the advantage of also strengthening the leg joints, including hips, knees, and ankles. Because it involves closed-chain work encompassing multiple muscles and joints, it is considered excellent functional training. As the lower body becomes stronger through balance training, additional weight work can be added to help the upper body regain more muscular strength and endurance as well. It is at this point aerobic endurance training can begin, because the now added body symmetry and functionality will allow for endurance with less pain.

Aerobic endurance training needs modifications for those with FM. Some forms of this training will be easier than others. Minimizing eccentric muscle work, keeping the arms below shoulder level a majority of the time, and the ability to avoid holding one position for long periods are all important. Just as important is "starting slow and keeping it low." An often-advised frequency is for the new FM exerciser to begin at two times per week and advance very slowly to three or four times a week. When a flare occurs, altering workouts to short spans of exercise throughout each day might be a possibility, although waiting until the flare subsides might prove to be necessary. Exercise intensity is another concern. Aiming for 60 to 70 percent of maximal heart rate for twenty to thirty minutes is a good goal. While most FM exercisers will not want to start at this level, aiming for that goal while establishing a regular pattern of normal exercise can be motivating. Low-impact exercise such as outdoor or treadmill walking, reclining stationary exercycles, and water-therapy classes can be good choices for those with FM. Water workouts are often advised for chronic pain, but they can be problematic due to the natural resistance of water. A water fitness leader who understands how to reduce both eddy and frontal resistance (the drag that occurs when moving through water), and can program pauses into the workout, will help those with FM avoid postexertional fatigue.

In step classes, boot camp classes, and martial-arts-style classes the norm is performing repetitive movements or power combinations, and the likelihood of muscle fatigue and joint stress is increased. These exercise workouts are not optimal for FM. Dizziness and neurally mediated hypotension (low blood pressure and lightheadedness linked to fainting) are common complaints in FM patients. Neurally mediated hypotension may appear during prolonged standing or in response to physically stressful situations. For individuals with these co-morbidities, care must be taken to avoid quick turns during movement workouts.

Workout sessions that last longer than thirty minutes are not necessary for those with FM and can actually produce diminishing returns. Delayed Onset Muscle Soreness (DOMS) is a legitimate concern with chronic pain, and specifically for those with FM. It can be prevented during workouts by limiting deep lunges and squats and avoiding endurance-repetition challenges. It is also important to note that the typical endorphin release experienced by the general population is often not present in chronic pain exercisers. This group may go many months before exercise typically begins to feel good.

Diet

People with FM are very interested in what dietary changes they can make to minimize their symptoms. Diet is something within the patient's control and rational changes are encouraged by clinicians. Fad diets are not recommended for those with FM. These include liquid, single-food, high-fat, high-protein, or low-carbohydrate diets. Fad diets are also sometimes touted for specific diseases. An example is an arthritis diet that avoids nightshade vegetables. There is no researched evidence of symptom relief in this diet for either FM or arthritis.

Although several dietary studies have been done in FM, there is no single FM diet. Instead, helpful dietary changes encompass two goals: to optimize health with the same recommendations given the general population and to treat FM co-morbidities affected by diet. These co-morbidities include obesity, celiac disease, lactose intolerance, and irritable bowel syndrome.

Obesity is treated by portion control, by identifying the behavioral stimuli leading to overeating, and by choosing healthier food options. Two studies on obesity in FM are noteworthy. One used a Weight-Watchers-type approach by employing a daily food diary and weekly body weighing. Participants noted significant weight loss and symptom reduction. In a more invasive study intervention, persons with FM and morbid obesity underwent gastric bypass surgery. Twelve months later, after losing an average of 90 pounds per subject, study participants were significantly less symptomatic. It must be noted that FM should not be suspected of being an offshoot of obesity. While many persons with FM are overweight, this is most likely due to the necessity of limiting activity levels that are part of coping with the disorder. Further, studies looking at body mass index against symptom severity do not demonstrate a relationship between weight and FM symptoms. Indeed, people with very low body mass indices like that found in anorexia nervosa (an eating disorder characterized by extreme weight loss and body image distortion) also can have FM. Incorporating a healthy diet to further optimal health is important for everyone with FM, not just the overweight person. In summary, obesity should be treated, since it is associated with myriad other health problems, and it has been demonstrated that weight loss may reduce FM symptoms in obese FM patients.

Celiac disease is a genetic autoimmune condition where certain grain-based products are harmful to the body. An inflammatory response becomes evident in the lining of the intestines and produces abdominal pain, fatigue, and, sometimes, abdominal distention. A series of blood tests followed by a small bowel biopsy can confirm the presence of celiac disease. If present, a referral to a registered dietitian is in order, as many prepared foods contain hidden sources of grains that will need to be eliminated from the diet.

Lactose intolerance (sensitivity to milk sugar) is very common. It is not thought to be overrepresented in FM, but it can be missed due to the prevalence of GI pain in FM. Reporting a challenge from dairy-based products is considered diagnostic without further lab tests being necessary. Many substitution products contain an enzyme to reduce abdominal bloating caused by the kind of internal gas related to lactose intolerance. Other measures include reducing or eliminating dairy from the diet. Some persons with lactose intolerance find that liquid dairy products are more problematic than solid or semisolid dairy products.

The dietary intervention that has shown the most promise thus far in FM is called The Living Foods Diet. This diet consists of fresh fruits and vegetables and unrefined grains. Those with FM who could tolerate the strict nature of the diet demonstrated improvement in multiple FM symptoms. Excitotoxins are molecules (such as MSG and aspartame) that can lead to neurotoxicity when used in excess. In 2001, another peer-reviewed case study involved a challenge elimination diet. Four subjects with FM who removed dietary excitotoxins from their diet reported a reduction of symptoms when the products were removed and a return of symptoms when the products were placed back into the diet. It may be possible that The Living Foods Diet has been successful in part due to elimination of the food additives described in the case study. A study is under way now investigating a controlled challenge/elimination diet in persons with FM and irritable bowel syndrome. Foods being eliminated in this study will include the types of packaged foods that often contain excitotoxins, including flavored potato chips, seasoning packets for dehydrated noodles, most canned soups and broths, most fast foods, soy sauce, and various seasoning salts.

A variety of unusual vitamins, herbs, and nutraceuticals have been touted to cure FM, but it is the mainstream vitamin products used to improve general health in everyone that can be considered worthwhile as treatment options. Vitamin deficiencies do need to be treated; for example, vitamin D deficiency is very common in FM. Vitamin D is measured in the blood, and clinicians typically recommend over-the-counter vitamin D, although they may write a prescription depending on blood levels. Similarly, vitamin B-12 may need to be measured in patients who have numbness and tingling in their extremities. Vitamin B-12 or combinations of the B vitamins may be indicated if selected blood markers are low. Magnesium has muscle-relaxing properties and may be helpful for some people with FM. Occasionally, magnesium is given intravenously (directly into a vein) and mixed with vitamins, a procedure called "Myer's cocktail." Other agents such as blue-green algae and Fibronol (a supplement containing ocean-based products) have not been demonstrated to be effective in rigorously controlled double-blind studies.

Complementary and Alternative Therapies

Many persons with FM turn to providers of complementary and alternative medicine (CAM). CAM providers are consistently ranked highly by FM patients. Unfortunately, the studies on the efficacy of CAM therapies in FM are somewhat inconsistent. Nonetheless, many patients experience relief from alternative medicines, and CAM treatments can be considered additionally helpful in restoring hope and confidence for the future; this outcome should not be minimized. The fine line to be negotiated when selecting CAM therapies is protection for finances when recommended therapies include benign but costly ineffective or untested treatments. Alternately, persons who have tried CAM therapies with no relief may feel guilty for not improving. A stellar CAM provider, like a stellar allopathic (standard Western medicine) provider, will reassure patients that if therapies are not effective it is not the patient's fault. Continuing to use and promote an unproven therapy that shows no ongoing health advantage to the patient is always unacceptable in any practice of medicine. Well-tested CAM therapies for FM include acupuncture, chiropractic, electrical therapies, and various vitamins, herbs, and nutraceuticals. Although their mechanisms of action have yet to be fully elucidated, they may be due in some part to stress reduction and their ability to elicit the relaxation response. Patients also might learn to elicit the relaxation response without involving a CAM provider if these therapies prove helpful. Self-help techniques include deep breathing, meditation, central focus (single focus on a word like a mantra or object), and progressive muscle tensing and relaxing.

Acupuncture (a technique of inserting and manipulating fine needles into specific points on the body to relieve pain) was demonstrated to be beneficial in initial open-label studies, meaning that there was no control group. Later, randomized, placebo-controlled studies failed to demonstrate a significant symptomatic improvement but did show objective improvement findings with neuroimaging (body-scanning technology). Some CAM providers have argued that "sham acupuncture points" cannot be a true placebo. Others state that traditional Chinese medicine is not easily studied using allopathic standards, since treatments are not standardized but are individualized to the patient and acupuncture is usually combined with herbal therapies. Acupuncture will continue to be tested in FM, particularly in its connection to the correction of autonomic dysfunction (malfunctioning of the nervous system). One study did demonstrate significant improvements by using electro-acupuncture. It is thought electro-acupuncture may work by releasing tight fibrous bands and muscular contraction knots, similar to the way dry needling (injecting a solid needle into a pain site) or tender-point injections (numbing agents injected into a pain site) are thought to work.

Chiropractors are very useful in FM as they often make the initial diagnosis. This may be due to patients seeking chiropractic manipulation after whiplash-type injuries. Some chiropractors report their adjustments in FM patients do not "hold" like in non-FM patients, and, to date, there is no evidence to support chiropractic adjustments are helpful in the treatment of FM. However, the role of chiropractors may take place early on by diverting regional pain so that it does not become widespread pain, and thus avoiding a leap to central sensitization, the precursor of FM.

Electrical therapies and magnet therapies are frequently used by people with FM, with highly varying levels of success. While there is no evidence reporting magnet therapy to be helpful in FM, electrical therapies have displayed a role in pain relief. Prior to understanding the chemistry of synaptic exchange (specialized junctions through which neurons signal to each other), electrical therapies were common. Nowadays, medications are more commonly used to alter synaptic exchanges, and electrical therapies have fallen into disuse. The FDA has approved certain electrical devices for the treatment of recalcitrant depression. None have been approved for the treatment of FM. Painless stimulation through the scalp or earlobes are the most common therapies. Further study is needed to know if these will be helpful for people with FM. An older, better studied electrical therapy is the Transcutaneous Electrical Nerve Stimulation (TENS) unit, most commonly used for chronic back pain.

Overall, many therapies both pharmacologic and nonpharmacologic play an important role in the treatment of FM. Since coping with chronic illness is a life-long journey, persons with this disorder can and should take advantage of the many options available for symptom relief and quality of life enhancement. Scientists continue working hard to understand the causes of FM, and their future results will make it possible to fine-tune symptom relief within a multitude of treatment options.

6

Common Co-Morbidities

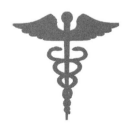

There are multiple co-morbidities (associated disorders) that commonly coexist with FM. Some of these are diagnosable diseases within themselves, whereas others are not considered a separate disease but are considered symptoms. The connection between FM and the associated disorders that are considered symptoms is not yet fully understood. Overall, the common co-morbidities associated with FM are thought to be changes resulting from alternations (changes that occur in a successive manner) in the functioning of the autonomic nervous system (ANS) and the central nervous system (CNS). Many of these disorders are now called Central Sensitivity Syndromes because of their shared underlying pathophysiology, especially due to the findings in brain neuroimaging (images that show the structure or functioning of the brain, such as a CAT, SPECT, PET, or fMRI scan).

The eleven commonly recognized co-morbidities we discuss in this chapter include: chronic fatigue immune dysfunction syndrome, irritable bowel disorder, irritable bladder disorder, chronic headaches, temporomandibular joint dysfunction, Restless Legs Syndrome, pelvic pain syndromes, multiple chemical sensitivities, mood disorders, cognitive dysfunction, and cold intolerance.

Chronic Fatigue and Immune Dysfunction Syndrome (CFIDS)

In the U.S. population, 0.5 percent of people meet the criteria for CFIDS, compared to 5 to 15 percent of the population who are diagnosed with FM. The overlap between the two shows that 35 to 70 percent of those with CFIDS have FM, whereas 20 to 70 percent of those with FM report an additional diagnosis of CFIDS. Earlier terms for CFIDS included *yuppie flu* or *chronic Epstein-Barr Syndrome*. CFIDS is defined by the Centers for Disease Control as a medically unexplained, persistent, or relapsing fatigue that is not substantially alleviated by rest and which is associated with significant functional impairment, including fatigue that occurs concurrently with four of more of the following: cognitive dysfunction, sore throat, tender lymph nodes, muscle pain, joint pain without swelling, headaches, lightheadedness, unrefreshing sleep, and postexertional malaise lasting for at least twenty-four hours. These symptoms must persist at least six consecutive months to be diagnosed as CFIDS. As there is no simple test to confirm CFIDS, diagnosis is based on history and physical exam. Tests are often done to rule out other diseases that might mimic this syndrome. These may include blood testing for thyroid dysfunction, hepatitis B and C infection, Lyme disease, syphilis, along with occult stool tests (fecal sampling that detects bowel cancer) and a CBC (complete blood count). Occasionally people with neurodegenerative diseases like multiple sclerosis are temporarily misdiagnosed with CFIDS. The cause of CFIDS remains only partly understood, but alterations in the ANS and CNS are pathophysiologic changes that have been seen. More recently, immune and inflammatory markers are being studied. Treatments are symptom-based and include both drug and nondrug therapies for fatigue, depression, insomnia, cognitive dysfunction, pain, dizziness, and lightheadedness.

Irritable Bowel Syndrome (IBS)

IBS is one of the most common co-morbidities in FM, affecting 30 to 80 percent of FM patients. Previously, IBS has been known by names such as "irritable colon," "spastic colon," nervous indigestion, and functional colitis. Sometimes IBS is predominated by constipation, at other times by diarrhea, but it can also occur as constipation alternating with diarrhea. Symptoms include chronic constipation or frequent diarrhea associated with abdominal pain, tenderness, bloating, and gas. Sometimes symptoms are exacerbated by meals or stress and relieved by bowel movement. A smaller percentage of patients also have nausea, vomiting, and loss of appetite. Additionally, pain from bowel stretching is amplified by central sensitization. Although the pathophysiology is not completely understood, some believe that the syndrome is associated with altered gastrointestinal mobility and permeability. Fortunately, there is agreement that IBS is not associated with structural problems in the bowel and does not progress to autoimmune inflammatory bowel diseases (IBD) such as Crohn's and ulcerative colitis. Diagnosis is made by history and physical exam. Blood tests or imaging such as endoscopy (a medical procedure used to assess interior surfaces by inserting a tube into the body) are performed to rule out other problems such as colon cancer or IBD. Treatments are rather hit or miss, requiring patients to try a variety or combination of treatments. These may include various diarrhea and constipation medications, anticholinergics (drugs that eases muscle contractions), tricyclic antidepressants, dietary change to add fiber, peppermint oil, reducing food additives and caffeine, and a recommendation to exercise.

Irritable Bladder Syndrome (IB)

IB has gone by many names including irritable bladder syndrome, overactive bladder, idiopathic bladder spasm, and "detrusor instability" (detrusor is the medical name for the bladder muscle). Of all people with FM, 5 to 50 percent are thought to have IB. In this syndrome the bladder suddenly contracts, even without being full. These contractions cause an irrepressible need to urinate, medically termed *urgency*. IB causes urination frequency, meaning that people often have to urinate seven to ten times daily and often during the night as well; a medical term for this is *nocturia*. Embarrassingly, urge incontinence occurs in about half of the persons with IB. This is urinary leakage before the patient can reach the toilet. The cause of IB is not known, but miscommunication in the neurological system is the prime suspect. The neurological link is further supported by the prevalence of IB following a stroke or in persons with Parkinson's disease. Diagnosis is made by history and physical exam. If a urinalysis indicates blood in the urine, then imaging studies will be done to rule out any malignancy or other disease pathology. Treatments are aimed at reducing the symptoms and gradually training the bladder not to respond until it is closer to full. This is called bladder training. Bladder training is sometimes aided by the use of a TENS unit, placed suprapubically. Pelvic floor exercises, called Kegels (*KEE-gulls*), are encouraged as well. Other treatments include providing a bedside toilet for nocturia with urgency, decreasing caffeine, alcohol, sodas, and fruit juice to see if those may be triggering symptoms, and monitoring quantity of fluids intake. Medications include anticholinergics and antispasmodics (drugs that eases muscle contractions and spasms) to block nerve impulses and relax the bladder. Dry eyes and dry mouth are common side effects of these medications. Tricyclic antidepressants, selective serotonin and norepinephrine reuptake inhibitors, and antihistamines also may be helpful.

Chronic Headaches

Chronic headaches occur in 3 to 5 percent of adults worldwide. And at least 25 percent of people with FM experience chronic headaches, with chronic migraines and chronic tension headaches being most common. The definition of chronic headache is a headache that occurs at least fifteen days per month for three or more months. Symptoms will vary depending on the type of headache.

Chronic migraines usually affect one side of the head and are characterized by pulsating, throbbing, severe pain. The headache can be aggravated by physical activity, bright light, and loud noise. Sometimes nausea and vomiting also occur during migraine headaches. Chronic tension headaches usually start as intermittent headaches, typically involve both sides of the head, and are mild to moderate in severity. They have a band-like pressure or squeezing quality. Diagnosis is made by history and physical exam. Imaging studies and spinal fluid analyses may be done if brain injury, infection, or tumor is suspected. A newer theory explaining the relationship between these two types of headaches is called the convergence theory. Basically, the convergence theory proposes that chronic tension headaches are simply aborted migraine headaches and that these two types of headaches are more closely related than previously thought. Treatments depend on the type, frequency, and severity of the headaches. Drug treatments include antidepressants, beta blockers, anticonvulsants, triptans (such as Imitrex and Amerge), and NSAIDs. Some people with FM have headaches in response to taking too much pain medication; these are called rebound headaches. Sleep deprivation, stress, and skipping meals also may trigger chronic headaches.

Temporomandibular Joint Dysfunction (TMD)

TMD was previously called TMJ syndrome. The temporomandibular joint allows the lower jaw to move up and down and side-to-side, to enable talking, chewing, and yawning. Symptoms of TMD include pain that moves through the face, jaw, or upper neck. Muscles feel stiff and the joint itself may lock, click, or pop. In the United States, 10 percent of the population will seek professional treatment for TMD, whereas 75 percent of people with FM are thought to have TMD. This dysfunction's onset may be caused by jaw trauma, infection, some types of arthritis, or bruxism (chronic grinding of the teeth). In a best-case scenario, TMD is self-limiting; in other cases it will need ongoing treatment that may include deep heat, ultrasound, a soft-food diet, the avoidance of chewing gum, and the application of ice packs. Severe cases of malocclusion (misaligned teeth or a poor lineup between the dental arches) may require an orthodontist who can provide specialized dental work that will prevent teeth from breaking. Interestingly, orthodonture (preventing and correcting irregularities of the teeth) recently has been identified as a risk factor for TMD.

Restless Legs Syndrome (RLS)

RLS and its closely associated cousin, periodic limb movement disorder, cause jerking movements intermittently throughout the night, typically every twenty to thirty seconds. In the United States, 3 to 15 percent of the general population is thought to have RLS, whereas 30 to 60 percent of people with FM report the same set of symptoms. Symptoms include an irresistible urge to move the legs, sensations of creeping, crawling, numbness, itching, tugging, and tingling. These symptoms tend to become worse during prolonged sitting or at night and improve when the legs are moved. Severe RLS can also involve the arms and even the trunk. RLS is thought to be occasionally associated with attention deficit disorder (ADD) and commonly occurs with end-stage renal (kidney) disease dialysis. The diagnosis is based on history and physical exam, and sometimes a sleep study will be ordered to check for other sleep disorders, such as sleep apnea. For those whose RLS disrupts or prevents their sleep, medications used to promote sleep might include anticonvulsants, benzodiazepines, opioids, and dopamine agonists. People who do not respond to treatment with sleep medications also may benefit from iron, B-12, and folic acid supplements. Pregnant and perimenopausal women are at higher risk for RLS due to iron deficiency. Nonpharmacologic agents may be used in conjunction to prescription and over-the-counter medications and include reducing or eliminating alcohol from the diet, walking, stretching, and massage or acupressure before prolonged inactivity. Some people report RLS relief with marijuana, but clinicians do not commonly recommend this. A number of oral canabanoids are under study that are hoped to work similarly to marijuana without its euphoric side effects (see www.clinicaltrials.gov). Some medications, including antihistamines, antiemetics, tricyclic antidepressants, and certain antipsychotics can worsen or actually cause RLS.

Pelvic Pain Syndrome (PPS)

Known PPS diagnoses include:

Endometriosis: Growth of endometrial cells in a location outside of the uterus.
Dysmenorrhea: Painful uterine contractions in the lower abdomen during menstruation.
Vulvodynia: Chronic burning, stinging, irritation, or rawness of the female genitalia.
Vulvar Vestibulitis: Painful inflammation of small glands at the entrance to the vagina.
Prostatodynia: Painful inflammation of the prostate.

PPS affects one in seven women in the United States and a smaller proportion of men. These syndromes are overrepresented in FM, with reports that at least 20 percent of persons with FM also have PPS. This group of disorders can be defined as pain for three consecutive months that localizes to the anatomic pelvis and causes functional disability sometimes requiring surgery. The diagnosis is made based on history and a physical exam, and tests may be ordered to rule out infection, malignancy, postoperative complications, and referred pain from other locations or disorders. Ruling out other factors is important, since in FM chronic pelvic pain also may be related to abdominal wall myofascial (*my-oh-FASH-ee-al*) trigger point pain, chronic pain postures, hernias, and irritable bowel syndrome. The pathophysiology of PPS remains unclear, but abnormal pain processing is consistently noted on neuroimaging studies. Treatments include pain medications, tricyclic antidepressants, and anticonvulsants. Topical treatments are used in vulvodynia and vulvar vestibulitis.

Dysautonomia

Known dysautonomia diagnoses include:

Postural Orthostatic Tachycardia Syndrome: Faintness and racing heart in response to prolonged motionless standing.

Neurally Mediated Hypotension: A steep drop in blood pressure after prolonged motionless standing, sometimes including nausea and visual changes.

Vasovagal Syncope: Fainting from a change in body position, commonly lying to standing.

Mitral Valve Prolapse Syndrome: Chest pain, palpitations, agitation of uncertain cause.

Joint Hypermobility: Abnormally increased mobility of small and large joints.

Marfan Syndrome: Genetic disorder of the connective tissue with ANS and cardiac involvement.

Dysautonomia is the term used to describe diseases and malfunctions of the autonomic nervous system (ANS). ANS pathways in the brain and the nerves serve to regulate the vital functions of the body and maintain homeostasis (the body's ability to remain stable in the face of change). The primary symptoms that present in patients with dysautonomia are excessive fatigue, dizziness, vertigo, panic, and rapid changes in heart rate. In earlier times women with dysautonomia were diagnosed with *neurasthenia*, a psychopathological term first used to describe symptoms.

The prevalence of dysautonomia in the general population is unknown, but it is common in FM. Symptoms include severe fatigue, syncope (*SINK-a-pea*) (loss of consciousness), near-syncope (falling down to faint but not losing consciousness), cognitive dysfunction, and heart racing during prolonged standing. Tests used to identify dysautonomia include heart rate variability testing and tilt table tests. Treatments are dependent on which specific dysautonomia diagnosis is found. Treatments may include increasing salt and water in the diet, wearing compression stockings, avoiding sudden changes from supine (lying down with the face up) to standing, and avoiding prolonged standing. Treating dysautonomia can be a trial-and-error process since a treatment that helps one individual may actually worsen the symptoms of another.

Multiple Chemical Sensitivities (MCS)

MCS is one of the least understood co-morbidities associated with FM. MCS previously has been termed *toxic injury, chemical injury syndrome, twentieth century syndrome, sick building syndrome, idiopathic environmental intolerance,* and *toxic-induced loss of tolerance.* Due to alterations in the central nervous system, all people diagnosed with FM are more sensitive to light, noise, smell, and pain. MCS, however, is a more pronounced, debilitating chronic sensitivity to low levels of chemicals or other substances in industrialized society. The most common offenders include smoke, pesticides, plastics, synthetics, petroleum products, and paints. Symptoms are multisystem and can include runny nose, itchy eyes, scratchy throat and scalp, headaches or earaches, sleep disturbance, GI symptoms, cognitive dysfunction, difficulty breathing, and skin rash. A cause for suspicion of MCS occurs when an individual is exposed to a sensitizing agent and improves or resolves completely when the triggering chemicals are removed. The clinician will then diagnose MCS based on history and physical exam. It is important to rule out illnesses with similar symptoms such as panic disorder, dysautonomia, allergies, and thyroid dysfunction. Treatments include eliminating all offending substances from the surrounding environment. This often takes years, since the following are often found to be the offending agent or agents: food dyes, petroleum products, smoke, agricultural chemicals, cleaning fluids, volatile organic compounds, glues, paints, bleach, fabric softeners, laundry detergents, perfumes, air fresheners, scented candles, hair-care products, and even highlighter markers. Fortunately, there is no evidence of a long-term buildup of toxic chemicals in the body or an increased early mortality associated with MCS. No medications have been consistently demonstrated to be effective for most people with MCS.

Mood Disorders: Depression, Anxiety, Posttraumatic Stress Disorder

Depression, anxiety, and posttraumatic stress disorder (PTSD) often coexist and are generally called "mood disorders." Thirty percent of people with FM are currently depressed and 60 percent have a lifetime history that includes a depressive episode. There are several subtypes of depression, each having a slightly different clinical presentation and treatment. Generally, depression is diagnosed based on a history of feeling down, sad, blue, hopeless, guilty, anxious, or fatigued. Besides mood changes, there are often changes in eating and sleeping patterns, all of which can interfere with daily life and normal functioning. As with most chronic illnesses, there is no single known cause of depression. Instead it is thought to be caused by a combination of genetic predisposition, environmental factors, and environmental triggers that alter biochemistry. There is a preponderance of evidence from brain-imaging technologies demonstrating consistent brain alterations compared to people without depression. Specifically, the parts of the brain responsible for sleep, appetite, behavior, and mood are affected. Neurotransmitters such as serotonin and norepinephrine also are out of balance, and neurotransmitters are a key to optimal communication between nerve cells.

Therapy for depression includes prescription medication combined with talk therapy. Cognitive behavioral strategies largely have replaced psychoanalysis in the treatment of mood disorders. The main key to success in treatment appears to be early and adequate intervention. Drug classes for depression include tricyclic antidepressants, SSRIs, SNRIs, and occasionally monoamine oxidase inhibitors (MAOIs). However, MAOIs have multiple drug and food interactions. Occasionally, stimulants or anti-anxiety medications are used in conjunction with antidepressants. Exercise, electrical therapies, and light therapy are all helpful in some types of depression.

Depression is a major risk factor for suicide, and suicide is the leading cause of premature death in FM. Types of depression include: major depressive disorder, dysthymic disorder (a low-grade, chronic depression), postpartum depression, psychotic depression, and seasonal affective disorder. Bipolar disorder previously was called manic depression but is not technically a form of depression. A diagnosis of depression is made by patient-reported history. Physical exam and laboratory tests may be done to rule out thyroid or other endocrine disorders, viruses, and other medical issues.

Anxiety is a symptom that may include physical or psychological feelings of distress and worry, changes in heart rate, skin temperature, and myriad other features. Generalized anxiety disorder (GAD) is an anxiety disorder that presents as excessive, uncontrollable, and often irrational worry about everyday problems for at least six consecutive months. This worry limits people's ability to work, go to school, and function in the community. People with GAD are more symptomatic than people with anxiety as a symptom. They may anticipate disasters, exhibit catastrophic thinking, have fatigue, fidgeting, headaches, muscle aches, trembling, sweating, and insomnia.

PTSD is an extreme anxiety disorder that is disabling and exhibits permanent neurological changes. Although an estimated 50 to 90 percent of people encounter some trauma over their lifetime, only about 8 percent will develop full-blown PTSD. It can either appear after a person encounters a single traumatic event or ongoing terrifying experiences, such as military combat, natural disaster, or violent attack. The encounter that triggers PTSD can either take place when the individual is the prime victim or when witnessing a traumatizing experience. High predictors for developing PTSD include childhood trauma, chronic severe adversity, and high family stress. PTSD is commonly treated using a combination of psychotherapy and medications. Drugs used to stop panic attacks also may prove useful in reducing the impact of traumatic memories.

Cognitive Dysfunction

Cognitive dysfunction, sometimes called fibro-fog, is common and highly distressing in FM. Cognitive changes include difficulty with short-term recall, speed of thought processing, verbal fluency, and multitasking under distraction. There is evidence that these deficits are consistent with healthy persons who are at least twenty years older than the person with FM. There is no evidence that fibro-fog will progress into dementia, Alzheimer's, or Parkinson's disease. Nonetheless, cognitive declines do interfere with the ability to remain gainfully employed at a level consistent with education. Loss of full-time employment often means significant income reduction that is often followed by a lack of health insurance.

Cold Intolerance

Most people with FM report cold intolerance. This may or may not relate to autonomic dysfunction in the form of cold-induced vasospasm. Before treating cold intolerance, primary providers need to rule out vascular and autoimmune illnesses. Treatments then include wearing nylon or other sweat-retaining clothing under regular clothes, using ice tongs rather than hands when retrieving ice, and wearing gloves in the grocery store to access refrigerator and freezer sections. Aerobic exercise also may work to improve temperature regulation. Conversely, high-dose beta-blockers such as propanalol may be associated with cold hands and feet.

In summary, readers will note that many of the co-morbid conditions described here have similarities in pathophysiology, especially neuroimaging. Likewise, the treatments for many of these conditions can be similar. It is easy to understand how patients with FM might be placed on multiple medications in an attempt to manage not only FM but its common co-morbidities. This speaks volumes to the general public who might wonder why one disorder requires so much time and money. But it is plain to see now that complicated illnesses do indeed require complex resources.

7

Cultural Impact

Adjusting to life with FM will mean redefining expectations for self, family, vocation (work), and avocations (hobbies). Financial changes often occur, including the loss of full-time income and health insurance, so filing for disability or worker's compensation often becomes a necessity. In fact, it has been shown that 26 percent of people diagnosed with FM are on disability. The cognitive behavioral treatments listed in Chapter 5 are helpful in the transition to accepting FM and living optimally with it. Following are five practical strategies gleaned from patients who are thriving in spite of their FM.

First, individuals with FM must learn to accept that there will be unanticipated ups and downs. Life with FM is sometimes two steps forward, one step back. Overscheduling will lead to a fibro-flare, but sometimes there is no apparent reason why a flare suddenly occurs. Being prepared mentally both for the results of overdoing it and also for unexpected flares can save the individual from blaming themselves or dwelling in self-pity. Instead, a positive approach can be taken, concentrating on good self-management of the flare or strategizing ways to avoid overscheduling in future. Over time, people with FM also learn that flares do eventually subside and better days lie ahead.

Second, those with FM must focus carefully on what might trigger a flare and keep track of diet, exercise, travel, mediations, and family changes. Often overlooked flare instigators can include even positive changes, like vacations, parties, and other pleasurable pursuits. Journaling not only makes unsuspected flare triggers apparent but also gives patients the opportunity to read about times they were doing better. During a bad flare this can help to remind them that not all days are terrible. Journaling is empowering and helps people ride out a flare by recognizing temporary setbacks and leading away from catastrophizing. Measuring and recording good days is great self-therapy.

Third, those with FM need to find pleasurable distractions and incorporate them into their lives. Distraction from pain is a key coping strategy. Intellectual pursuits may provide a distraction and also give people a feeling of accomplishment. Being engrossed in a hobby helps some people refocus their energies away from their distress and toward the task at hand rather than staying absorbed by their symptoms. Laughter is also a wonderful distraction, and can come from interacting with children, watching silly movies, and reminiscing about old times.

Fourth, the individual with FM will need to consciously select a positive life attitude. Optimism and pessimism are personality traits, and they are also a decision. How one views the world and their disorder can become more optimistic. Choosing to be optimistic helps people feel less dependent on others and gives hope for the future. Some people with FM have found that volunteering to help people with other conditions, like blindness, provides an opportunity to feel thankful and optimistic. For others, the altruism of participating in a FM research study may promote optimism by helping the next generation of people who will be diagnosed with FM. Participating in research can really be thought of as a form of living philanthropy.

Fifth and finally, learning to love one's new self is essential to functioning optimally. This is a hard process since the United States rewards productivity and, very often, quantity over quality. Re-creating oneself is an up-and-down task that will involve trial and error. One key is to avoid a list of "shoulds." If the inner voice says: "I should be able to do this" or "I shouldn't have to stop now," it only promotes guilt and negative thinking. Instead, individuals can make a list of things they can do. Eventually, reviewing the list of all of the things that are possible will provide a list of realistic goals that can be turned into accomplishments. Many therapists tell patients with chronic illnesses to never "should on themselves." The bad joke usually brings a laugh but underneath is a telling truth.

Chronic illness redefines the individual, their family, and friends. Using the practical five steps mentioned earlier may help people live more optimally. Eventually science will catch up with FM, and people will not need to work so hard to maintain some semblance of normality and quality in their lives. This has been demonstrated in illnesses like depression, asthma, and gastric ulcers. As treatments improved, people with these chronic conditions were able to focus more on life and less on their illness.

Following is an interview with a young woman with FM whose name is Amy. As you read through her interview, observe carefully her discussion of the impact of FM on her life, and how it mirrors the information you have read in this book.

Her personal story and her plan for the future also demonstrate the journey toward an optimal quality of life undertaken by many individuals with FM.

Amy's Story

1. **When did you first notice the symptoms of FM?**

   It's difficult to know for sure because I've had health problems all my life, especially in the last ten years. But I noticed some changes in my symptoms about a year ago in 2008 and began to suspect I had fibromyalgia.

2. **What concerns did you have about your symptoms before you learned it was FM?**

   I think the scariest symptoms were the cognitive problems. I was starting to feel like I had dementia or something! Also, before a diagnosis there was always a worry in the back of my mind that something really serious might be wrong, like cancer or Lou Gehrig's disease.

3. **How did your family, friends, and acquaintances respond to your symptoms?**

   My short-term memory problems had myself and some of my friends teasingly calling me Blondie. For my family, the fatigue and pain were the harder symptoms to deal with because they limited my activities so much, both the fun stuff and especially work and housework. Though my mom didn't say it, I think it was hard for her not to see my fatigue as just laziness on my part. She told me I needed to learn how to deal with it and go on with normal life activities.

4. **Who diagnosed you? Did you see many different providers before getting a correct diagnosis?**

   My older sister was diagnosed with FM many years ago, so at least I knew enough to eventually ask to be checked for it. Even so, I didn't get diagnosed right away. I saw a naturopath for years and was able to get some help but never completely resolved the problems. I complained to my primary-care doctor about my insomnia and pain levels, and she referred me to pain and sleep clinics without attempting to find out what might be the base cause of those problems. A nurse from the pain management class at the sleep clinic finally referred me to another doctor who diagnosed me with FM.

5. **How did your family, friends, and acquaintances respond to your diagnosis?**

   They were happy for me, as strange as it sounds. Most of them understood how important it was to me to know why I was experiencing my health issues and to have a "label" so that my doctors would have an idea of how to help. I did have a couple of friends who weren't familiar with the word *fibromyalgia*. One of my friends told me that a mutual friend had asked her if I was going to die. In an effort to help them understand, I made a webpage about fibro and how it affected me personally, and I think they appreciated that.

As soon as I had an official diagnosis, my family began to be more understanding of my need to pace, rest, and not do certain things like vacuuming because they would raise my pain levels too much. I know in some ways it was hard on my parents, though, because it's hard for them to see me unhealthy. I am the youngest in my family, and now all of their children have been diagnosed with a chronic illness. But having sisters who also have invisible diseases means we can understand each other and support each other in a deeper way. My parents are great at doing what they can to help out, too.

6. **What other associated disorders (the co-morbidities like CFIDS, Restless Legs Syndrome, etc.) of FM do you experience?**

   I have IBS, occasional migraines, and Raynaud's. Not associated with FM, I also have a vision-related learning disability and recently found out I have some heart problems, possibly a complication of the Raynaud's.

7. **How has FM affected your schooling, your friendships, your recreational activities?**

   The college program I am in is difficult even for healthy students. I'm training to be a sign language interpreter, which means cognitive processes and physical movements are vital. I've failed several tests because I happened to be having a fibro-fog day with almost no short-term memory or was having language production problems. Also, when I'm sore and stiff, I can't sign as clearly or as long. Of course, fatigue and concentration problems can make homework a challenge. However, God has given me His strength to succeed, and overall I'm doing pretty well in school—I certainly couldn't do it on my own! Most of my teachers have been really understanding, too.

   I've had to cut back a lot on recreational activities and hanging out with friends and family. Last fall I went on a short hike with some friends and almost ended up in the ER from the pain. My friends are great. They know that I can't do a lot of activities and that often even if I am planning on getting together, I sometimes will have to cancel at the last minute because of pain or fatigue. I've found Internet connections like email, instant messaging, and Facebook to be a low-stress way to get in some social time with friends when I'm not up to going out. A quiet night chatting or watching movies is nice, too.

8. **What changes have you made that really help you cope with symptoms?**

   Emotionally, I think the most important change I made was a viewpoint change. I went from thinking of myself as sick to thinking of myself as disabled. As I mentioned, I've struggled with health problems for many years. During that time I always saw myself as sick. A person who is sick will get well (or die). There is an end to it. I lived thinking this was a temporary setback and that when I was better I would be able to do such-and-such. Each time I was feeling better, I would get hopeful and think this time I was finally getting well. When inevitably I began to feel sick again, it would be a bit depressing.

About a year ago, even before I got the official diagnosis, I came to the realization that I was never going to get completely well. I went through a time of mourning and shed a lot of tears. Then I was able to accept it and the limitations it brought and move on. I have learned to live the best life I can, and not sit around and wait "until I'm well" or get lost in focusing on the things I can't do. When I have bad days I keep my spirits up by reminding myself that soon I will have a better day. It's also helped to see how God has been able to use my experiences to allow me to reach out to other people that otherwise never would have let me in.

Physically, the most important change is learning how to pace and letting it be okay that I can't do everything. I'm learning how to say no and how to ask for help, whether that is asking a friend to carry my backpack for me, asking the government for a disabled parking placard, or going to the disability office at my school.

9. **What are your own plans and hopes for the future? How has FM contributed to those plans?**

   I'm a freelance writer and have many ideas for books and stories I want to write. I think FM has given me empathy for those who are suffering and has given me a deeper appreciation for life. These are things that make my writing stronger, and I am able to touch more people with my writing as a result.

   I am also planning to be a sign language interpreter. I'm hoping to graduate and start part-time work in a few months. It's a little bit harder to see how my FM contributes positively to that, because the symptoms can interfere so much. But on the other hand, I know the empathy I've gained and my appreciation of having to struggle to do things the world calls "normal" will help me connect even more to my deaf clients.

10. **What's the main thing (or things) you wish more people understood about FM?**

    I think the hardest part of FM to understand is the fibro-fog. For one thing, not very many people are aware that it exists. When I mention FM, most people respond with, "Oh, that's the thing where you hurt a lot, right?" or "Oh, that's the thing that makes you tired all the time?" Few people seem to understand the full scope of all the FM symptoms. When I do try to explain fibro-fog, I hear dismissive things like, "Oh, I forget what I'm saying in the middle of sentences sometimes, too." It's hard to explain how severe and confusing it can be.

I think it can also be difficult for people to realize how much FM fluctuates, both in the vast differences between each person that has it and the day-to-day symptom changes. Sometimes, something I can do one week will cause severe pain another week.

It's also important for people to understand that even on the days when a person with FM looks good and seems to be functioning well they are still experiencing some pain and other symptoms. And more than likely, even if they can get through the day okay, when they get home they crash.

HOPE FOR A CURE

Chronic illnesses are chronic simply because, as yet, there is no cure. An acute illness like strep throat used to be chronic or even deadly because scientists had not isolated the bacteria causing the illness and had not developed the antibiotics to cure the illness. In the past scarlet fever, which is a consequence of strep throat, was a death sentence for millions. Now, it is just an inconvenient day away from work and school and a trip to the pharmacy. More recently, gastric ulcers were a cause of significant lifelong suffering. Patients were told to reduce stress in their lives, and this sometimes included quitting their jobs and leaving their families. They also were encouraged to avoid spicy foods and drink more milk. All of these therapies were largely ineffective. In some cases, people with long-standing gastric ulcers died from the bleeding in their gastrointestinal tract. In the late 1900s, a cure was found. Now people with gastric ulcers take a breath or blood test, followed by a round of medication, and are often permanently cured. A final example is HIV disease. In the early 1980s, HIV was a death sentence, with the individual's demise often coming within a year of diagnosis. Now, although HIV cannot yet be cured, a combination of long-term medications can keep the infection and many negative consequences at bay for decades.

Like scarlet fever and gastric ulcers, fibromyalgia will someday be a temporary inconvenience, and people will be able to regain their normal health after prompt diagnosis and appropriate treatments. The purpose of this discussion is to remind readers that initially many chronic illnesses are met with suspicion and patients blamed for their illness. They are often treated with stress reduction until the disorder is better understood by scientists and adequate treatments are readily available to clinicians.

The hope for a cure, or at least a long healthy life free from many FM symptoms, is now realistic goal. Three decades of objective, reproducible laboratory abnormalities have built the foundation for testing therapies. Scientists are currently testing how both *pharmacologic* and *nonpharmacologic* therapies improve the objective pathophysiology in FM. The object findings consist largely of neuroimaging (brain and spinal cord visualization), cytokine or chemokine dysfunction, autonomic nervous system changes, muscle abnormalities, and a host of HPA axis changes. Another route toward a cure often comes from clinicians and patients acting on trial and error.

The hope for a cure for FM is real. It is not yet known if the puzzle will be brought together by clinicians, patients, or scientists. Most likely, it will be a combination of these people, working in concert. Science, unlike industry, is largely open and free. Discoveries continue to be made available through peer-reviewed publication, and thanks to the Internet, people around the globe can learn from others' findings, building new theories and testing new therapies. The scientific literature then grows exponentially and hope for a cure becomes a tangible possibility rather than merely a dream.

Appendix A

Treatment Stories

MEDICATIONS IN CLINICAL PRACTICE

The following is an alphabetized listing of drugs often used in treating fibromyalgia with symptoms, with comments on typical dosage and use. *Not tested in fibromyalgia

Common prescription terms used:

bid = twice daily
hs = at bedtime
q = every
qd = every day or once daily
qid = four times daily
sub-q = subcutaneous
tid = three times daily
transdermal = skin delivery (typically a patch)
transmucosal = oral delivery (typically under the tongue)

Medication generic/trade: Alprazolam / Xanax
Clinical pearl: This medication has an extremely short half-life. It may not be suitable as a through-the-night sleep aid if taken earlier in the evening, at bedtime.
Common dosage: 0.25 to 3 mg a day

FM usage: Panic attacks, anxiety, or early morning awakenings

Patient example: Mary is a 31-year-old female who grew up in an abusive home environment. Even though she is safe now as an adult, she has found she sometimes has nightmares that leave her heart racing and body sweating, and she is unable to go back to sleep after awakening around 4 a.m. Alprazolam was prescribed for sleep and anxiety by her psychiatrist. She takes one around 4 a.m. on the nights she awakens from a bad dream. Alprazolam, in concert with cognitive behavioral strategies, allows her to go back to sleep for another two to three hours. With this combination, she is able to remain employed full-time and raise two young children with the help of a supportive husband.

Medication generic/trade: Amitriptyline / Elavil

Clinical pearl: This is the most-tested drug agent prescribed for FM. Its use is well-supported by meta-analyses published recently in JAMA (Journal of the American Medical Association).

Common dosage: 10 to 50 mg at hs in a single dose

FM usage: Mild pain, sleep

Patient example: Rob is 55 years old, semiretired, and works in the construction industry. He has had numerous work-related accidents over the past thirty-five years. Fortunately, none required hospitalization or surgery. He does, however, have mild FM, sleep-onset insomnia, TMD, and IBS. He also has a history of alcohol and drug abuse, although he never required hospitalization or rehabilitation. He has not had a drink or used drugs for more than two decades. He makes sure none of his prescribed medications are potentially habit forming. His primary-care provider wisely chose Amitriptyline, 25 mg at bedtime, knowing that it would help him fall asleep. He manages his daytime pain with physical therapy, cognitive behavioral strategies, and NSAIDs. The constipating side effects of Amitriptyline worked in his favor due to his diarrhea-prone IBS. He has been able to remain employed and is now working as a contractor, a position that fortunately allows him to keep health insurance since self-employment insurance was more than $1,500 a month.

Medication generic/trade: Apo-zopiclone

Clinical pearl: This medication is the precursor of Lunesta. It is only available by mail-order through Canada. It tested well in an FM randomized, controlled research trial.

Common dosage: 7.5 mg at hs

FM usage: Sleep

Patient example: Florinda is a 38-year-old female whose FM flares when she has insomnia for more than three consecutive nights. Her FM onset began shortly after her first child was born nine years earlier. She had noticed a gradual onset of low back pain and difficulty sleeping. She and her primary provider wrote off these symptoms to the typical demands of caring for a new baby. Now both of her children are in elementary school, and none of her friends have the same amount of pain and disrupted sleep that Florinda still endures. She saw a rheumatologist because she thought she might have lupus and was diagnosed by the rheumatologist with FM due to her widespread pain and tender points on physical exam. Lupus was ruled out based on a negative history of sun-exposure rash, nonelevated liver or kidney enzymes, no history of fluid around her heart or lungs, or other signs common in lupus. She also had a negative ANA and normal sedimentation rate. She tried Amitriptyline first but found she gained weight, had difficulty thinking clearly and multitasking, and experienced dry mouth and constipation. She now orders Apo-zopiclone from Candadrugs.com. Her doctor gives her a prescription for three months, which she faxes to the Canadian Web site. A pharmacist at the Web site contacted her for a medical screening, and the medication was later mailed to her. The Canadian medication works particularly well for Florinda because, although she has medical insurance from her part-time job, she does not have prescription drug coverage. She also uses Tramadol during the day as needed for pain. This combination has improved her symptoms by 50 percent. She enjoys her children again and doesn't endure the long sleepless nights anymore.

Medication generic/trade: Bupropion Hydrochloride / Wellbutrin*
Clinical pearl: This medication may be prescribed to augment SSRIs
Common dosage: Slow release 150 to 300 mg SR bid or 300 XL qd
FM usage: Depression, anxiety, fatigue, fibro-fog
Patient example: Michela is a 28-year-old female graduate student with a long-standing history of mild depression and intermittent anxiety. She smokes two packs of cigarettes a day to help cope with her anxiety. She was diagnosed with FM last year, and her pain is 30 percent better with Pregabalin 250 mg bid. However, her mood was not improving. Her psychiatric mental health nurse practitioner (PMHNP) knew that Bupropion was helpful not only for mood but for smoking cessation and encouraged Michela to continue the Pregabalin and add Bupropion. As her mood symptoms improved, her PMHNP started a smoking cessation plan. Although quitting was very difficult and required five attempts, Michela can now sleep through the night without waking from a nicotine craving. Overall, her FM is about the same, but she is sleeping better, has improved mood, and is looking forward to graduation this spring.

Medication generic/trade: Carbidopa, Levodopa / Sinemet*
Clinical pearl: Inexpensive
Common dosage: 10/100 to 20/200, 1 tab hs
FM usage: Restless Legs Syndrome
Patient example: Lawrence is a 62-year-old male who has had FM since a minor motor vehicle accident two years earlier. His sister has had FM for nearly

thirty years. In addition to aches and pains, Lawrence notices that he avoids long car trips or air travel. He even avoids going to the movies or to church. He reports that all of these activities make his legs hurt or sometimes feel like something is crawling on them. He finds he must stand up and walk around to relieve the sensations. Further, at night he has great difficulty going to sleep because these symptoms also occur when he is in bed. His provider diagnosed him with Restless Legs Syndrome. The provider first changed his short-acting opioid to Tramadol to see if that was precipitating the restless legs. The good news was that Tramadol was effective for his pain without the constipating side effects of many opioid medications, which he now only uses for a flare. The bad news is that the restless legs continued. Iron and vitamin B blood tests revealed no problems, so his provider prescribed Carbidopa, one hour before bedtime or prior to prolonged sitting. Lawrence's restless legs improved by 75 percent, and his life has become a little more normal. He no longer avoids activities that require prolonged sitting, sleeps better at night, and was able to attend his grand-daughter's two-hour-long ballet recital without discomfort.

Medication generic/trade: Carisporodol / Soma*
Clinical pearl: This medication is taken only at bedtime if it has previously caused daytime fatigue.
Common dosage: 350 mg, one to four times per day
FM usage: Muscle relaxation, pain, sleep
Patient example: Rinda is a 56-year-old female who has FM but complains that muscle stiffness is her most limiting symptom. After a battery of tests to rule out other causes of muscle and joint problems, her provider determined that her muscle stiffness was due exclusively to FM. In addition to Duloxetine, her base-line medication for FM, she has tried Flexeril, Zanaflex, Robaxin, and NSAIDs. None have helped the stiffness. Her provider prescribed Carisporodol at bedtime and further prescribed a low-dose exercise program. Rinda's stiffness is much improved, and her story showcases the "trial-and-error" approach that is often necessary in FM. Many medications have to be tested before a good combination is found for each individual patient.

Medication generic/trade: Clonazepam / Klonopin, Clonapam*
Clinical pearl: In one author's opinion (KDJ), this drug is one of the best adjuncts for sleep in FM.
Common dosage: 0.25 to 2 mg hs, tabs or quick-dissolving wafer for faster onset of action and potentially lower total dosing.
FM usage: Anxiety, Restless Legs Syndrome, sleep
Patient example: Vicki is a 40-year-old nurse who has had aches and pains for the past decade. She initially attributed them to injuries from moving patients and to prolonged hours standing on her feet for twelve-hour shifts. She thought

her sleep problems were due to working swing shifts and also wondered if maybe she was experiencing early menopause. Her primary provider diagnosed her correctly with FM. They spent the next year working on cognitive behavioral strategies, exercise programs, physical therapy, and sleep hygiene. She gave up working swing shifts, even though that meant a slight reduction in pay. Her sleep and pain improved about 30 percent, but she was still unable to fall asleep or sleep for more than two hours despite trying the three FDA medications approved for FM and a plethora of over-the-counter sleep aids, including Benadryl and melatonin. She could not tolerate Zolpidem due to nightmares and sleepwalking. Her mother, who also has FM, told Vicki that she had been taking a low-dose of Clonazepam for nearly thirty years without dose escalation or tolerance. Vicki reported this to her provider who agreed to have her try Clonazepam. One year later Vicki's sleep is 75 percent improved and she remains employed full-time. She is able to take a very low dose due to her strict adherence to good sleep hygiene measures.

Medication generic/trade: Cyclobenzaprine / Flexeril
Clinical pearl: This drug is almost identical to Amitriptyline in structure.
Common dosage: 5 to 30 mg at hs
FM usage: Muscle relaxation, mild pain, sleep
Patient example: Chad is 30-year-old former professional soccer player. Although he never had a serious head or neck trauma while playing soccer, he had to give up the sport after a third knee injury requiring surgical repair. He thought the aches and pains he had endured over the past decade were a result of playing a contact sport with an "aging" body. During his convalescence, however, he realized something different was happening. Chad's knee was healing beautifully and his primary provider, an orthopedic surgeon, was not sure what to do for Chad's continued pain. He referred Chad to a physiatrist who specializes in sports medicine. At that point, he was diagnosed with FM. Chad was uninsured at the time since he was in the midst of changing careers, so the costly FDA-indicated medications for FM were out of reach for him. The physiatrist recommended an old medication, often marketed as a muscle relaxant. Chad tried Cyclobenzaprine 10 mg tid. While his pain and stiffness were much improved, he felt groggy and couldn't think clearly during the day. Now he just takes the medication at bedtime. Fortunately, the restorative sleep he had been missing seems to also be helping his daytime pain.

Medication generic/trade: Dextromethorphan
Clinical pearl: Side effect is "out of body" feeling.
Common dosage: 30 to 120 mg in twenty-four hours
FM usage: Pain, weak NMDA receptor agonist. Adjunct to Tramadol with or without acetaminophen (Ultram / Ultracet) before moving to scheduled narcotics.

Patient example: Wilson is a 44-year-old administrative assistant with multiple drug sensitivities. He has had FM since his early 30s after contracting an unknown viral illness during an international trip. Pain is his primary limiting FM symptom. Wilson is one of the few people with FM who does not have sleep difficulties. Tramadol brings his pain down from seven out of ten to five out of ten. He tried a variety of short-acting narcotics, but all caused extreme nausea and skin rash. For Wilson, the side effects of the narcotics were not worth the added improvement in pain relief. Wilson's provider tried multiple other medications, but none were terribly effective. A rheumatologist who was working down the hall from Wilson's primary provider shared an abstract reported at a scientific meeting. The abstract reported that Dextromethorphan, an ingredient in cold medications, could be prescribed alone and was thought to act on pain pathways. Wilson's provider discussed this with Wilson, who said he was willing to try anything in order to reduce his pain and keep his job. Fortunately, the Dextromethorphan has not caused nausea, vomiting, or skin rash, and Wilson's pain has been reduced. His pain scores are lowered now to four of out ten.

Medication generic/trade: Dicyclomine, Hydrochloride / Bentyl*
Clinical pearl: This medication is both inexpensive and well-tolerated.
Common dosage: 20 mg oral qid
FM usage: Irritable bowel syndrome/pain
Patient example: Lucinda is a 32-year-old woman with long-standing constipation-prone IBS. Recently she was diagnosed with FM. Interestingly, she has tried no medication for either her IBS or FM. After a history, physical exam, and laboratory tests ruled out both IBD (inflammatory bowel disease) and lactose intolerance, her provider asked if she was more concerned about the IBS or the FM. Lucinda reported she felt IBS limited her life more than FM. The provider prescribed Dicyclomine and peppermint oil and referred her to a registered dietitian who helped Lucinda start a gradual dietary program to reduce food additives, especially MSG and aspartame. They gradually have added fiber and increased her water intake. After six months, Lucinda's IBS is at least 50 percent improved. She says she was not aware how much she relied on fast foods and now cooks at home 90 percent of the time. She states she is now ready to explore treatment options for her FM.

Medication generic/trade: Duloxetine Hydrochloride / Cymbalta
Clinical pearl: This drug needs to be taken with food to decrease the common side effect of nausea.
Common dosage: 20 to 120 mg per day
FM usage: Depression, sleep, pain
Patient example: Caroline is a 51-year-old account executive. Over the past couple of years she has noticed increasing back, upper arm, and hip pain. She

also reports that she tosses and turns all night and feels fatigued during the day. She attributes these symptoms to a stressful job in an uncertain economy and perhaps also the start of menopause, although her periods are still normal. Her gynecologist tested her hormone levels and found they were all within normal range. She was given the alpha-blocker Clonodine, 0.5 mg at bedtime, and that helped her fall asleep, but it did not help her to stay asleep. Further, it did nothing for her pain. A rheumatologist confirmed that she had FM, but he did not want to manage her symptoms, as he preferred to care for people with rheumatoid arthritis, lupus, and other autoimmune diseases. Her primary provider was not familiar with FM treatments but knew that Duloxetine was recently approved for the treatment of FM whether patients have concurrent depression or not. He had Caroline start as the Duloxetine package insert suggested, at 30 mg with breakfast. After a few weeks he increased the dosage to 60 mg. Within two weeks, Caroline's pain and fatigue improved by 30 to 40 percent. Most importantly, her confidence has returned. She states she feels "in control" again, and she has now started a gentle exercise program. She also is relieved she didn't have a more serious, life-threatening disease and has not had to quit her job. She did, however, have brief counseling regarding pacing and boundary-setting at work and home. She practices these techniques fervently since she does not want to return to her previous poor health status.

Medication generic/trade: Eszopiclone / Lunesta*

Clinical pearl: This medication is the precursor of Zopiclone and is indicated for long-term use.

Common dosage: 2 to 4 mg at hs

FM usage: Sleep

Patient example: Paula is a 44-year-old medical social worker. Through her work she has seen what it means to be sick and has observed firsthand the health consequences of losing one's job and medical insurance. So last year when she began having difficulty sleeping, she immediately employed the stress reduction and sleep hygiene techniques she teaches to her clients. She does have aches and pains but not enough tender points to technically meet the criteria for the treatment of FM. Because of her job, Paula is well aware which providers in her town are most knowledgeable about the treatment of FM. Her provider urged her to do "whatever it takes" to sleep well so she does not progress to full-blown FM. After feeling "hung over" after several weeks of taking Amitriptyline at night and having no success with calcium, magnesium, B-vitamins, St John's Wart, or melatonin, Paula elected to try generic Zolpidem 10 mg. She found it amazingly helpful, but after four hours of wonderful sleep, she was unable to go back to sleep for the rest of the night. She discontinued the Zolpidem and switched to Eszopiclone 3 mg taken one hour before bedtime. For the past six months, she has enjoyed seven hours of uninterrupted sleep each night and now has more energy and concentration during the day. Her aches and pains have improved 50 percent, and she has only an occasional tender point now on exam. While she would prefer not to take any medications, she understands the importance of sleep in keeping her potential FM at bay.

Medication generic/trade: Ethyl Chloride, Fluorimethane® spray termed Spray and Stretch*

Clinical pearl: Trochanteric bursitis is sometimes mistaken for the greater trochanter trigger point and is effectively treated with local steroid injections.

Common dosage: Dependent upon body region affected and severity

FM usage: Muscle pain and myofascial pain syndrome

Patient example: Bob is a 55-year-old sales executive who travels from Los Angeles to New York weekly. He always intends to exercise at the hotel but finds himself checking his email and taking clients to dinner instead. Although he sleeps well and denies daytime fatigue or poor mood, he does have "painful knots" in his muscles. He went to a chiropractor and a massage therapist a couple of times and found relief, although it generally just lasted for a few hours. He eventually spoke of his muscle pain with his primary provider who confirmed that he had myofascial pain syndrome. He warned Bob that this could progress to FM if left untreated. Bob was surprised, as he has always thought of FM as a "woman's disease." Bob accepted a prescription for Ethyl Chloride, had it filled at the pharmacy, and took it with him to the physical therapist. There he learned how to stretch with the cooling spray. An occupational therapist also gave him an exercise routine he could do in airports, on airplanes, and in hotel rooms. While Bob is not happy he has to "pay attention to his health rather than his job," he is thankful that he can find relief through spray-and-stretch and exercise. At date of publication, Bob has not developed any new symptoms and does not meet the criteria for FM.

Medication generic/trade: Fentanyl Citrate / Actiq*

Clinical pearl: Due to potential side effects, it may be wise to limit the use of this medication to six months.

Common dosage: 200 mcq transmucosal

FM usage: Irritable bowel syndrome/severe pain

Patient example: Lynne is a 51-year-old former advertising executive who is now on workplace disability due to severe FM, IBS, TMD, and headaches. She takes six daily medications for these disorders and has four additional medications she can use on an as-needed basis. She is visiting her primary provider today after an emergency department visit over the weekend. The emergency department visit was necessary for stitches in her eyebrow area. The laceration above her eye occurred when she fell off the toilet and nearly passed out due to severe gut pain from IBS. Her provider gave her a prescription for Fentanyl

Citrate, three per month to use for severe pain. They also reviewed her IBS treatment plan and made more dietary modifications.

Medication generic/trade: Fludrocortisone / Florinef*
Clinical pearl: Patients who are suspected of having neurally mediated hypotension need to have the diagnosis confirmed with a tilt table test.
Common dosage: 0.1 mg
FM usage: Adjunct to treating neurally mediated hypotension, common in patients with fatigue and nausea that are greater than pain.
Patient example: Tristin is a 19-year-old woman who has had episodes of feeling lightheaded and dizzy for the past five years. She notices these feelings when she has to stand in long lines to buy tickets or groceries or when she waits for the bus. She also has a history of severe "growing pains" in her extremities. Now that she is finished growing, she isn't sure why the pain persists. She has been experiencing extreme fatigue and has elected to take a year off before beginning college to work on her health. Her pediatrician referred her to an internal medicine physician who ordered a tilt table test after ruling out myriad other causes for her dizziness, fatigue, pain, and near-syncopal episodes. At that point, she was diagnosed with neurally mediated hypotension. Initially, she was treated by increasing salt and water in her diet and wearing compression stockings which Tristin referred to as "old lady hose," although she found she could conceal them easily under her jeans. She tried to avoid prolonged motionless standing but found it could be difficult in the course of living her normal life. Finally, her internist referred her to an endocrinologist who initiated a low-dose course of a hormone called Florinef. Tristin noticed almost immediately that her daytime energy and concentration improved. Her near-syncopal episodes have become less frequent and severe. She is currently applying to colleges near her home and continues working with her internist on the overall management of her FM.

Medication generic/trade: Sodium Oxybate / Xyrem
Clinical pearl: This is a prescription-only medication that is only available directly through a central pharmacy. The FDA has approved Xyrem for excessive daytime sleepiness and cataplexy associated with narcolepsy.
Common dosage: 4.5 to 6 mg at hs, repeat three to four hours later if needed
FM usage: Sleep, fatigue, and pain
Patient example: Emily is a 55-year-old schoolteacher who has had FM for more than twenty years. She states that her pain is bearable but that her insomnia and daytime fatigue are making her consider taking an early retirement. This is problematic, not only because she needs the income, but also because she is still too young for Medicare coverage. The Cobra insurance option through her school district will cost her more than $800 per month. She has tried more than twenty different medications and myriad nonpharmacologic therapies. Many

have provided some relief but also brought with them a host of side effects. Six months ago she became a subject at an academic medical center that is researching Sodium Oxybate, a new medication being investigated for the treatment of FM. The medication is currently used for sleep disorders and excessive daytime sleepiness, but in earlier FM studies it has proved helpful for pain and fatigue. The academic researchers and clinicians explained that Sodium Oxybate appears to repair the deep sleep deficit that was discovered three decades ago to be present in those with FM. In order to enroll in the study, Emily had to discontinue all her other FM medications under the university doctor's supervision and abstain from drinking alcohol during the study. She agreed to "wipe the slate clean and try a new approach." After six months, Emily was randomized into the open-label portion of the Xyrem study and is now receiving the active drug at 4.5 mg rather than the placebo. She continues to receive the medication free of charge but returns to the academic center on a regular basis to report any potential side effects and provide information about her symptoms. She says that her sleep has improved 75 percent as has her fatigue. She also states her pain is now manageable, and she feels no need for other pain medications. She likes the fact that she is only on one medication and is hopeful that in the future this helpful agent will be indicated by the FDA for the treatment of FM.

Medication generic/trade: Gabapentin / Neurontin*
Clinical pearl: May cause daytime fatigue. Many patients take only an hs dose.
Common dosage: 900 to 3600 mg a day in two or three divided doses
FM usage: Neuropathic pain
Patient example: Martin is a 71-year-old man who has had chronic back pain for forty years along with peripheral neuropathy (painful sensations in his lower legs and feet) from diabetes for twenty years. He recently was diagnosed with FM. His nephrologist (a kidney specialist) diagnosed him with FM, which she was able to do because many of her other patients with end-stage renal disease who have gone on dialysis from diabetes also have FM. She consulted with Martin's internist who elected to try Gabapentin, a medication option available through the Veteran's Administration, the organization that is Martin's medical provider. Martin's overall FM and his peripheral neuropathy improved 30 percent in only six weeks. His interdisciplinary health-care team is now strategizing on how to optimize his health through a combination of pharmacologic and nonpharmacologic therapies.

Medication generic/trade: Growth Hormone (e.g., Nutropin)
Clinical pearl: This drug is not covered by third-party payers unless a patient has concomitant adult growth hormone deficiency syndrome.
Common dosage: Values dependent on serum Insulin-like Growth Factor levels and body weight. Daily sub-q injections are required.

FM usage: Depression, fatigue, pain, quality of life, exercise tolerance

Patient example: Marilyn is a 48-year-old endocrinologist. She has had FM for at least fifteen years. Recently, she had to reduce the scope of her medical practice to office hours only; giving up nights and weekends of being on-call. This significantly reduced her income and effectively eliminated the possibility that she could become a full partner in her group's medical practice. As an endocrinologist, she is a hormone expert. She has kept abreast of the growing body of literature regarding abnormalities in the part of the brain that prevents the adequate release of growth hormone. She contacted the study team who published randomized controlled clinical trials of growth hormone injections in FM to learn more about their current research findings. After following her low levels of IGF-1 (a long-term marker of growth hormone) for several years, she and her doctor decided to try growth hormone therapy. She first had a growth-hormone-stimulation test using a standard trial of Arginine and growth-hormone-releasing hormone. The test was normal, indicating that her pituitary gland would be able to release adequate growth hormone under a targeted pharmacologic stress. She began the daily injections and noticed very little improvement for three months despite her blood levels of IGF-1 normalizing within two weeks. She decided to persist, and within six months her sense of general well-being improved. Now three months later, her pain has begun to remit, and she has noticed that it is no longer as difficult to exercise. Fortunately, she has experienced no side effects like fluid retention or cardiac changes and plans to stay with the therapy long-term.

Medication generic/trade: Hydrocodone Bitartrate / Vicodin*

Clinical pearl: This medication is one of several short-acting narcotics. Many providers will move their patients to a long-acting medication when their patients use 90 to 120 tabs a month.

Common dosage: Varies with half-life of drug selected and pain level

FM usage: Moderate pain

Patient example: Thomas is a 60-year-old man with long-standing health problems. These include diabetes, Hepatitis C, heart disease including open heart surgery, and intermittent claudication (vascular pain in the legs). In the past he had a seizure, although the cause was never determined. He has twice survived cancer. The multiple illnesses, surgeries, and medications, including chemotherapy, have taken a terrible toll on Thomas's health. In the past year he has developed FM. Because he is on multiple medications for each of his other health conditions, his current goal is to reduce his pain from eight of out ten to five out of ten. He is not a candidate for Tramadol because of his seizure history. He is already on an anticonvulsant drug for his peripheral neuropathy. He cannot tolerate mood medications such as tricyclic antidepressants, SSRIs, and SNRIs. At his appointment with his provider, he was given Hydrocodone Bitartrate with a written handout discussing how to minimize constipation, fall risk, and the foggy thinking, all side effects from this medication. Two months later, his pain continues to be reduced and his quality of life is better.

Medication generic/trade: Lidocaine / Lidoderm Patch or Capsaicin Patch or Cream

Clinical pearl: Dry needling has been demonstrated to be somewhat effective for FM. However, in research acupuncture has not been consistently superior to sham points in FM.

Common dosage: Patch can be applied directly to FM trigger points or for back pain. Lidocaine can be directly injected into trigger points.

FM usage: Myofascial pain syndrome, regional pain, back pain

Patient example: Marilyn is a 56-year-old florist who has been diagnosed with FM and multiple chemical sensitivities for nearly two decades. Marilyn has tried twenty-seven different oral medications for FM but has been unable to tolerate the side effects. Fortunately, her major symptom is pain, with fewer problems regarding sleep, fatigue, and mood. Her job requires prolonged standing and unpredictable, intermittently long hours when large orders come into her shop. Her pain is managed almost exclusively with topical or injectable therapies combined with exercise, massage, and stress-reduction techniques. Marilyn uses an over-the-counter Capsaicin patch for back pain, a prescription Lidocaine patch for medial knee pain, Lidocaine injections, and ice and stretching for trochanteric bursitis (hip pain). With these therapies, she is able to remain employed and enjoy a reasonable quality of life.

Medication generic/trade: Loperamide / Imodium*

Clinical pearl: This medication is sold over-the-counter. Overuse can cause constipation. Providers might consider serum testing for celiac disease if considerable weight loss occurs.

Common dosage: 2 to 4 mg initially, up to 16 mg in twenty-four hours

FM usage: Mild diarrhea-prone IBS

Patient example: Lenore is a 32-year-old computer tech support staff person at a large call center. She has a college degree and loves helping her customers. Her FM is managed with Tramadol for pain and Clonazepam for sleep. She visited her provider seeking help for her diarrhea and abdominal pain because her symptoms have been becoming more frequent and severe, and they are interfering with her ability to work. Her provider tested her stool for infection and her blood for autoimmune GI illnesses. After a history and physical exam, he confirmed that diarrhea-prone IBS was the culprit. She started on dietary therapy for IBS and was advised to start with over-the-counter Loperamide. She was reassured that there were prescription antidiarrheal medications available if this was not adequate. She also received a letter from her provider to her employer asking for a work station near a bathroom for medical necessity. The employer was happy to comply, and Lenore is now able to continue to work comfortably and experiences less IBS symptoms.

Medication generic/trade: Lorazepam / Valium
Clinical pearl: The abuse potential for this drug was documented in the 1970s.
Common dosage: 2 to 10 mg up to qid
FM usage: Sleep, anxiety, muscle relaxation, Restless Legs Syndrome
Patient example: Barney is a 72-year-old retired accounts receivable clerk. He has had generalized anxiety disorder for years and has been on an SSRI for the past ten years without much relief. When asked when he last felt well, he replied that it was before the psychiatrist who prescribed Lorazepam for him for more than forty years died. His new psychiatrist thought that Lorazepam was not safe. Barney met the history and physical exam criteria for FM and, in fact, had probably had it for more than two decades. Moreover, he had symptoms consistent with Restless Legs Syndrome and no other illnesses or laboratory markers that could explain an alternative cause for his restless legs. He was titrated from an SSRI onto an SNRI and referred to a new psychiatrist. This new provider believes that his quality of life was superior on Lorazepam and feels comfortable restarting Barney on this medication. Two months later, his anxiety, restless legs, and overall FM are 50 percent improved.

Medication generic/trade: Methadone / Dolophine*
Clinical pearl: Patients may resist Methadone due to its use in heroin withdrawal.
Common dosage: 5 to 20 mg bid
FM usage: Moderate to severe chronic pain
Patient example: Juan is a 48-year-old man who was honorably discharged from the Marines after a combat-related head injury. He has myriad health problems including FM, panic disorder, chronic headaches, TMD, and dyscognition. Over the past fifteen years he has "climbed the ladder" of pharmacologic agents, not finding adequate relief with any of the medications he has taken. His Veteran's Administration insurance coverage includes Methadone, and in fact the center near his home has a chronic pain clinic for veterans. Juan has found support from an interdisciplinary team of health-care providers in the pain clinic and has now joined a support group of other veterans who have shared similar problems. Although he is still disabled, his quality of life has improved and he remains on a stable dose of Methadone to date.

Medication generic/trade: Modafinil / Provigil
Clinical pearl: Side effects of this drug may include headaches or insomnia. Case reports support its use in FM.
Common dosage: 200 to 400 mg q in the a.m.

FM usage: Severe daytime fatigue or fibro-fog

Patient example: Tina is a 24-year-old college student on medical leave who has chronic fatigue syndrome and FM. Multiple rounds of antibiotics and antiviral treatments at a Lyme disease clinic in her city have provided no relief. She also reports difficulty concentrating. She was diagnosed with attention deficit disorder (ADD) as a child but states that she "probably grew out of it." She says she does not experience sleep problems at night but mentions she has been falling asleep at inappropriate times during the day. Her health-care provider ordered a sleep study and a multiple sleep latency test (a test of excessive daytime sleepiness). She was found not to have a primary sleep disorder. She was offered Modafinil, 200 mg in the a.m., which she may repeat once midday, if needed. Six weeks later, she has no new symptoms such as headache or difficulty sleeping and her fatigue is 30 percent better. She has been working with a speech therapist regarding dyscognition. Her confidence in her cognitive abilities has improved significantly as well. She plans to start school in the fall.

Medication generic/trade: MS Contin / Kadian*
Clinical pearl: This medication should not be given to opioid–naïve patients.
Common dosage: 15 to 60 mg bid
FM usage: Moderate to severe chronic pain

Patient example: Mona is a 45-year-old woman who has had quite a tragic life. She had multiple adverse early life events. While trying to raise the family in a war-torn country, her parents were killed and she then experienced protracted abuse. She eventually moved to a neutral country, but it quickly became evident there would be lifelong consequences stemming from her physical and emotional trauma. Her provider diagnosed her with FM and sent her to a psychiatrist who worked in concert with a psychologist regarding her mental health. After years of non-opioid pain medications, short-acting opioids were tried. She quickly moved to 90 to 120 a month and was moved to longer-acting low-dose opioids. She is on Social Security disability and lives in a small home with eight other relatives who give her emotional support. She remains hopeful that newer pain medications will allow her to live a more normal life.

Medication generic/trade: Nonsteroidal anti-inflammatory agents (NSAIDs)
Clinical pearl: Overuse of this drug results in rebound headaches. It is of minimal relief for overall FM pain but works in decreasing peripheral pain generation.
Common dosage: Depends on agent chosen
FM usage: Chronic headaches, tendonitis, concurrent osteoarthritis

Patient example: Margo is a 71-year-old retired dancer. At one point, she was a prima ballerina and, later, the owner of a prestigious dance studio where she consistently worked six to seven days per week. Margo developed mild FM at the age of 65. Her most limiting symptoms are pain in her knees, feet, and ankles. Her provider examined her carefully and noted that she met the criteria for osteoarthritis of both knees but was not yet a candidate for joint replacement. She was also diagnosed with plantar fasciitis and ankle tendonitis. All three diagnoses possibly were due to the weight-bearing needs of her vocation. Although she had never had a GI bleed, her provider elected to use a cox-2 selective NSAID and Tramadol with Acetaminophen. He also injected her knees for osteoarthritis and referred her to physical therapy and to an orthotist for her plantar fasciitis and ankle tendonitis. Her knees were 50 percent better within two days of the injections. Her feet and ankles were better with orthotics and therapies. Decreasing these three major sources of peripheral pain generation also reduced her overall FM pain by 30 percent. She is very satisfied with her outcome.

Medication generic/trade: Oxycodone / Percocet, Percodan*

Clinical pearl: This drug is often considered when Hydrocodone is inadequately effective.

Common dosage: Varies with half-life of drug selected and pain level

FM usage: Moderate pain

Patient example: Pamela is a 43-year-old mother of two who is having a hysterectomy for severe pelvic pain and endometriosis. She has had FM for at least five years, but pelvic pain is her most debilitating symptom. Knowing that pelvic pain is a potent spinal cord sensitizer, her surgeon wisely elects to treat her pain pre-operatively with Oxycodone, infusing the surgical site with Lidocaine and working in concert with the anesthesiologist to protect her neck from hyperextension during the anesthetic administration and to minimize the time her arms are held away from her body during the procedure. Postoperatively, she is placed on an aggressive course of narcotics with a weaning schedule over four rather than two weeks. Six months later her pelvic pain is 75 percent improved and her FM is 50 percent improved. She no longer takes Oxycodone but does take milder nonscheduled medications and now participates in gentle exercise therapy. She is currently enjoying raising her school-age children.

Medication generic/trade: Oxycodone Hydrochloride / Oxycontin*

Clinical pearl: Users of this medication are told not to chew or break this or any long-acting opioid tablet.

Common dosage: 10 to 30 mg bid

FM usage: Moderate to severe chronic pain

Patient example: Jack is a 60-year-old truck driver. He has changed jobs recently because his left shoulder, back, and leg pain have made it impossible for him to make long hauls. Loading and unloading freight also has become increasingly difficult as he has had to contort his body during lifts to protect the areas of his body that were most painful. Fortunately, the retail chain for whom he has worked for the past forty years offered him vocational rehabilitation, and he now works in the warehouse tracking inventory. This job allows him to intermittently walk, sit, and stand but does not require lifting. His primary provider initially sent him to an orthopedic surgeon to investigate whether back surgery would reduce his symptoms. Unfortunately, a surgical cure was not possible, and the diagnosis that best fit Jack's symptoms turned out to be FM along with osteoarthritis of the spine. He had taken a variety of nonscheduled medications over the years, and for the past year he had added a short-acting narcotic three to four times daily to his regimen. The pain pills worked pretty well for the first two hours, then the pain was as severe as ever and Jack found he had to endure for another two to three hours until it was time to take another tablet. His primary provider has discontinued the short-acting narcotic and has put Jack on Oxycodone 10 mg every twelve hours. With physical therapy, his new job responsibilities, and a lower dose of a longer-acting narcotic, Jack is able to remain employed and his pain is reduced.

Medication generic/trade: Pramipexole Dihydrochloride / Mirapex

Clinical pearl: Pilot studies of this drug have found that high dosages, i.e., 4.5 mg, improve overall FM symptoms for many individuals but also require concomitant dosing with a proton pump inhibitor or anti-emetic. More recent concerns about excessive shopping and gambling have arisen.

Common dosage: 0.125 to 1.5 mg at dinnertime or divided between dinnertime and bedtime

FM usage: Restless Legs Syndrome at low dose and overall FM at high dose

Patient example: Marvin is a 61-year-old daytime security guard, who has been working for the same company for more than thirty years. When he sits or lies down to sleep at night, he gets uncomfortable feelings in his legs "like there is Coca-Cola in my veins." If he doesn't move his legs or walk, the discomfort turns to a deep-aching pain and superficial stinging pain. His primary provider ordered a sleep study, which was normal except for occasional periodic limb movement disorder, a condition often associated with Restless Legs Syndrome. Marvin's FM was fairly mild and stable and was being treated with Pregabalin for pain and Tylenol PM for sleep. Marvin's clinician discontinued the Tylenol PM to see if it was linked to the restless legs and increased his nighttime dose of Pregabalin to help with sleep. Both of these measures improved Marvin's restless legs by 30 percent. The clinician then added Pramipexole starting at 0.125 mg one hour before bedtime and slowly increasing the dose to .5 mg over several weeks, at which point the restless legs symptoms had abated. Marvin has been able to remain employed and has added some stretching exercises to his overall treatment plan.

Medication generic/trade: Pregabalin / Lyrica
Clinical pearl: One side effect of this drug is fatigue.
Common dosage: 450 mg divided bid
FM usage: Fatigue, pain, sleep
Patient example: Brittany is a 32-year-old mother of two who "feels like she is 60." She had a gradual onset of FM in her mid-20s and decided to leave the workforce despite having a graduate degree and working as a physical therapist. After her children were born, her FM significantly worsened. She had avoided medications over the past six years while she was trying to conceive or when she was pregnant or nursing. Now she would like to try medication with the primary goal of improving her sleep and reducing her pain. If possible, she would like to return to work at some point. She has specifically asked about Pregabalin, as she has seen advertisements for it on television. Her provider advised her that Pregablin was the first drug to be indicated for the treatment of FM by the FDA. In clinical trials it helped 30 percent of FM patients feel 50 percent better. More realistically, 50 percent of the patients felt 30 percent better. She was warned to start low and go slow with the dosing, so she started Lyrica at 50 mg at bedtime. To minimize the side effects of dizziness and sleepiness, each week she slowly increased her nighttime dose until she reached 225 mg. At that point she began an additional morning dose of 50 mg. She was satisfied with her symptom relief with a morning dose of 150 mg and an evening dose of 225 mg, despite the fact that the FDA indication was for 225 mg twice daily. Her provider has reassured her that her individual progress is more important than the goal dose. She has been able to implement a gentle exercise program and is incorporating the pacing she was taught by her physical therapist. She plans to return to work part-time in the next year when her children start preschool.

Medication generic/trade: Pyridostigmine Bromide / Mestinon
Clinical pearl: The medication provides improved anxiety, fatigue, sleep, and exercise ability but does not improve pain at rest.
Common dosage: 60 mg to 180 mg time span bid
FM usage: Normalize growth hormone response to exercise. May increase ability to exercise with less postexertional pain and fatigue.
Patient example: Jenny is a 47-year-old certified exercise instructor. Over the past five years she has noted feeling "worn out" after class and has experienced exercise-induced aches and pains that were taking longer to heal. Additionally, she was not sleeping as well at night. She had been diagnosed with FM two years earlier but was determined to "exercise my way out of it." She became interested in an article in a medical journal demonstrating that people with FM who exercise vigorously fail to produce a normal amount of growth hormone to repair muscle tissue. The study noted that the addition of Pyridostigmine 60 mg normalized the amount of growth hormone that patients made during vigorous exercise. Taking Pyridostigmine three

times daily for six months also helped sleep, anxiety, growth hormone release, and the ability to exercise. Jenny shared the article with her provider who agreed to prescribe the Pyridostigmine. She used it one hour prior to exercise and again at bedtime to maximize growth hormone release. Similar to the reported study results, she found that it was easier to exercise and her sleep improved. She eventually added a nonscheduled pain reliever during the day and was able to resume her usual exercise class teaching load. She also has retrained and has begun to focus on tai chi, warm-water exercise for elders, and gentle yoga classes.

Medication generic/trade: Roprinirole Hydrochloride / Requip
Clinical pearl: Used to treat overall FM symptoms; at higher doses this medication is limited in its use by side effects of nausea and dizziness.
Common dosage: 0.5 to 5 mg at dinnertime
FM usage: Restless Legs Syndrome
Patient example: Laura is a 62-year-old hairdresser who has been diagnosed with FM for nearly two decades. She is able to continue to work when she is able to get enough sleep. In the past her restless legs had been controlled with Sinemet. But over the past six months that drug seemed to stop working despite an increased dose. She also feels a dull ache in her right inner knee but without any cracking, swelling, or locking of the joint. Her provider carefully checked for peripheral neuropathy with electromyography studies and ran tests checking for adequate stores of iron and levels of vitamin B in her blood. All the tests were normal. A physical exam and X-ray of her knee also were normal. The provider replaced her Sinemet with Ropinirole 0.5 mg. Laura slowly titrated up to 2.5 mg but found it worked best if she took half that dose at dinner and the other half one hour prior to bedtime. Her restless legs symptoms abated, and her sleep improved dramatically as did her overall FM. She has been able to continue to work as a hairdresser, and she has followed the recommendation of her occupational therapist to invest in a well-cushioned floor pad to minimize the stress of the floor on her lower body. Her knee pain also remitted as she taught herself to turn her hairdressing chair with her hand rather than her knee—another alteration suggested by the occupational therapist.

Medication generic/trade: SSRIs (selective serotonin reuptake inhibitors). There are several in this class; those tested in FM include Fluoxetine, Citalopram Hydrobromide / Celexa, Sertraline Hydrochloride / Zoloft
Clinical pearl: Improvement in mood may not adequately treat pain and sleep disruption.
Common dosage: Depends on agent chosen
FM usage: Depression, Anxiety
Patient example: Mindy is a 36-year-old patient advocate at a local community center. Her clients are impoverished, and there is often little medical or

other support for them. As a result, her job is often frustrating and demoralizing. She was diagnosed with FM a year earlier after a whiplash-type injury morphed into widespread pain. Her sleep was very fragmented, but she continued to work because she was so much better off than her clients. When she finally consulted a physician about her symptoms, she broke down in tears. Instead of recognizing that the tears were from exhaustion due to lack of sleep, she was diagnosed with depression. As her doctor said, "Who wouldn't be depressed doing what you have to do all day?" She was placed on the newest, most selective SSRI to date. The selection was meant to minimize side effects. Unfortunately, it was of no help to Mindy. It is the older, less selective SSRIs like Fluoxetine that are more effective in FM. She eventually changed providers and tried an SNRI and was much happier with her symptom improvement. Mindy also has taken some of the same advice she gives her clients and coworkers about gentle exercise, stress reduction, pacing, setting boundaries, and planning enjoyable activities. Mindy still has FM, but she is much improved compared to a year earlier.

Medication generic/trade: Hydrochloride / Gabatril*
Clinical pearl: The side effects of this drug may include fatigue.
Common dosage: 4 to 56 mg a day given in two to four divided doses
FM usage: Neuropathic pain, sleep
Patient example: Emily is a 72-year-old homemaker who has had peripheral neuropathy of unknown origin for three years and FM for more than twenty years. Her sleep has become increasingly fragmented, and her Zonisamide / Zonegran is not helping her neuropathy as much as it did in the past. Her provider took a medical history and did a physical exam but found no indication of a new disease process. The provider decided to try a drug in a similar class that had been shown to increase time in deep sleep, although this was not its FDA indication. The provider discontinued the Zonisamide and replaced it with Gabatril. Emily now uses a higher dose of this medication in the evenings and a lower dose in midday. She is now able to enjoy the relief she experienced earlier with Zonisamide and is sleeping a bit more soundly as well.

Medication generic/trade: Tinzanidine Hydrochloride / Zanaflex
Clinical pearl: Individuals on this medication must have their liver enzymes monitored closely.
Common dosage: 4 to 8 mg hs
FM usage: Muscle relaxation, mild pain, sleep, stiffness
Patient example: Steve is a 66-year-old retiree and an avid gardener who was diagnosed with FM ten years ago. In the past year, Steve has noticed that his muscle stiffness is making it increasingly difficult for him to garden. His history,

physical exam, and diagnostic tests did not suggest osteoarthritis or a new cause for his muscle stiffness, so his provider elected to use Tinzanidine 4 mg at bedtime and 2 mg before gardening. Steve was an ideal candidate for this medication, as his liver health always has been perfect. A nurse at a local pain clinic made another suggestion for Steve so that he could continue gardening; she suggested he could go to a thrift shop and buy a few comfortable outdoor chairs and place them strategically throughout the garden. He could kneel on a knee pad and work his way toward a chair; then he could rest in that chair and enjoy viewing his work before starting on the next section. At first Steve thought this was a rather strange idea, but he decided to give it a try. Steve now has extended his garden by one-third, and his garden is now graced with four reclining vinyl chairs.

Medication generic/trade: Topiramate / Topamax*

Clinical pearl: This anticonvulsant is good for adjunctive pain management. Side effects can include fatigue and rash.

Common dosage: 25 to 100 mg

FM usage: Migraine prophylaxis

Patient example: Catherine is a 34-year-old woman who works from home by purchasing items from garage sales and then selling those items on the Internet. She has a college degree and used to work in the printing business, but the stress, lighting, and strong smells triggered her migraines and worsened her FM. She has had migraine headaches since her teens and was diagnosed with FM eight years ago. Over the past year, the frequency and severity of her headaches have increased and her migraine medicine is no longer aborting the headaches. A history and physical exam determined that migraine was still the correct diagnosis and that she would benefit from prophylactic therapy. This means she takes the medication every day and not just when she feels a headache coming on. Her sister had success for the same problem with Topiramate, so her provider decided to try the same therapy with Catherine, as genetics often determine how drugs are metabolized. Catherine's migraines returned to their previous rate, and she continues her online sales business to this day.

Medication generic/trade: Tramadol Hydrochloride with Acetaminophen / Ultracet

Clinical pearl: If individuals taking this drug can tolerate two tabs simultaneously, they may experience better pain relief.

Common dosage: 37.5 mg every four to eight hours not to exceed eight in twenty-four hours

FM usage: Mild to moderate pain

Patient example: Norma is a 41-year-old waitress who thought her aches and pains were due to job requirements. When she told her provider about her symptoms and added her further concern about her declining mood and poor sleep, she was diagnosed with FM. Interestingly, she now remembers that her grandmother had "rheumatism" and no one could hug her. Her provider elected to start her on Tramadol with Acetaminophen. When she returned for her follow-up visit, she mentioned that her symptoms were 20 percent improved and that she was having no side effects. Her provider then moved her to the following medication.

Medication generic/trade: Tramadol Hydrochloride / Ultram

Clinical pearl: This medication is a nonscheduled drug and has a low abuse potential. Providers will screen for seizure risk if they are prescribing a high dose in conjunction with SSRIs.

Common dosage: 50 to 100 mg every four to eight hours, not to exceed 400 mg in twenty-four hours

FM usage: Mild to moderate pain

Patient example: Because Norma could tolerate Tramadol with Acetaminophen without experiencing nausea, vomiting, or rash, the provider decided to try a stronger dose of Tramadol with no Acetaminophen. When her medication was changed, Norma noticed even more improvement in her symptoms. Meanwhile, her occupational therapist has given her multiple tips on how to alter her lifting and bending techniques in her job, and she has started a stretching program. Overall, Norma is now 40 percent improved from when she was first diagnosed.

Medication generic/trade: Transdermal Fentanyl (Duragesic Patch)*

Clinical pearl: All patients on chronic opioid therapy need to have constipation prophylaxis treatment.

Common dosage: 25 mcg/hr change q three days

FM usage: Moderate to severe chronic pain

Patient example: Belinda is a 50-year-old woman on disability due to a fall from a ladder at work. The fall resulted in a fracture to her spine and heel. Two back surgeries later, she was told that she had a phenomenon called "failed back syndrome." Since her surgeries she also had developed fragmented sleep, jaw pain (TMD), fatigue, and, understandably, depression. Belinda was doing better on an SSRI, but she could not tolerate any oral narcotics due to nausea and vomiting. She was given transdermal Fentanyl and multiple nonpharmacologic therapies. She has developed a new satisfying hobby, photography. This new hobby has entailed a steep learning curve, and the intellectual stimulation has proven to be a distraction from Belinda's unrelenting pain.

Medication generic/trade: Trazadone Hydrochloride / Desyrel, Trazon, Trialodine

Clinical pearl: The side effect of headache keeps some patients from using this agent.

Common dosage: 50 to 150 mg a day hs

FM usage: sleep

Patient example: Dora is a 55-year-old hotel shift supervisor who had prided herself on never missing a day of work despite often having to work overtime to help cover missed evening shifts due to employee shortages or sickness. Over the past year, Dora noticed that she was having increasing difficulty staying asleep, even though she initially was falling asleep instantly from what felt like exhaustion. She also developed a dull, aching pain in her neck, shoulders, and hips during this same time. After a thorough history, physical exam, and laboratory workup, Dora's health-care provider decided that her presentation most likely fit the diagnosis of FM. Because she was new to the diagnosis, the provider started conservatively with a low dose of nighttime Trazadone. Dora's sleep remained a challenge until she finally stopped working swing shifts and practiced multiple sleep hygiene therapies. Her employer was so happy with her performance that she was welcomed to a day-shift-only position. Dora was surprised by this, as she always thought that it was her "toughness" and work ability that made her valuable. It turns out that the quality of her work, rather than the quantity, was what her employer continues to value most.

Medication generic/trade: Zolpidem / Ambien

Clinical pearl: This is one of the most commonly prescribed sleep agents and is now available as a generic. Long acting Ambien is branded and dosed differently.

Common dosage: 10 mg hs

FM usage: Sleep

Patient example: John is a 52-year-old airline pilot who manages his aches and pains with NSAIDs and an occasional Flexeril. He had assumed his pain was due to being immobile for long periods of time and that his inability to sleep was due to multiple time zone changes. For many years, John used alcohol to help him fall asleep. Now the alcohol was no longer working. After visiting a sleep medicine physician and learning that his sleep study was normal, he sought the help of a primary-care provider. The provider encouraged him to consider using Ambien 10 mg, due to its short half-life. He also was sent to physical therapy to learn an exercise program he could use while on the road. Although he didn't have the necessary number of tender points to have the diagnosis of FM, it wasn't unreasonable to assume that he was headed toward the disorder. He was encouraged to completely avoid alcohol, which John had found unhelpful for his sleep anyway. John has been successful in incorporating an exercise program into his flight schedule and alternating between Flexeril and Zolpidem for sleep. He says he is actually starting to feeling better than he did ten years earlier before he began drinking alcohol.

Appendix B

The Fibromyalgia Clinic Questionnaire

When patients are evaluated for FM, the health-care provider needs a great deal of information about current and past medical problems. The Fibromyalgia Clinic Questionnaire, excerpted here, is a patient form that can be used to help health-care providers quickly and accurately evaluate people for the possible diagnosis of FM.

Because FM is more than pain, there are questions about physical functioning, mood, fatigue, sleep, restless legs, and other problems common in this population. An accurate assessment is the key to enacting appropriate clinical care.

FIBROMYALGIA CLINIC QUESTIONNAIRE

-Chronology of Problems-

Date of *onset* of FM symptoms:
Date of FM diagnosis:
Who first diagnosed FM?
The onset was related to which of the following (please circle):

An accident?	Y	N
An infection?	Y	N
An operation?	Y	N

Taking medications?	Y	N
Major stress?	Y	N
Toxic exposure?	Y	N
Other (describe below):	Y	N

Did you have pain "all over" from Day One?

If "*No*," how many areas were painful at onset?

Describe sites of *initial* pain (such as neck, left arm, etc.):

Are you right- or left-handed?

Have you ever had? (Please circle):
    arthritis, diabetes, high blood pressure, heart disease, osteoporosis,
    alcoholism, ulcers, kidney disease, liver disease, migraine,
    tuberculosis, stroke, psychiatric problems, epilepsy, lung disease,
    venereal disease, sciatica, drug dependency, thyroid disease, hepatitis,
    skin disorders, AIDS, fractures, multiple sclerosis, endometriosis,
    lupus, cancer, heart attack, carpal tunnel, breast implants,
    irritable bowel, Sjögren's, asthma, posttraumatic stress, sinusitis,
    vasculitis

Other diagnoses (describe):

Family History	Age	Health Problems	Living/ Deceased	Cause of Death
Father				
Mother				
Brothers				
Sisters				
Children				

How bad are your best and worst days of pain?
    Best days (0–10):
    Worst Days (0–10):

Please *check* symptoms below and indicate whether they are current or past:

Joint swelling	Poor sleep
Stiffness	Awaken feeling tired
Muscle pain	Restless legs
Muscle weakness	Hands change color in cold
Pain after exertion	Excessive fatigue for more than six months
Frequent headaches	Abdominal cramping
Chest pain	Constipation
Swelling or bloating	Abdominal distension
Difficulty swallowing	Intermittent loose stools

Daytime sleepiness	Frequent and urgent urination
Dry or itchy eyes	Impaired logical reasoning
Light headedness	Loss of memory
Depressed moods	Excessive anxiety
Breathlessness	Panic attacks
Dizziness	Premenstrual tension (PMS)
Impaired coordination	Tenderness of skin
Severe fatigue after exercise	Pain that keeps you awake

Other symptoms not mentioned above?

-Treatments-

Please list *all your current* medications:
List any drug allergies:

Have you ever been addicted to any drugs?

What past medications have you had? (*Circle all that apply*):

NSAIDS (e.g., Ibuprofen)	Opioids	Tranquilizers	Physical therapy
Ultram or Ultracet	Duloxetine	Pregabalin	Milnacipran
Antidepressants	Muscle relaxants	Gabapentin	Biofeedback
Sleeping pills	Injections	Exercise	TENS unit
Massage	Acupuncture	Steroids	Orthotics
Psychotherapy	Manipulation	Herbal meds	Chinese meds
Ambien	Diet modification	Surgery	
Others:			

List *medications* that have been of help:

List *nonmedicinal treatments* that have been helpful:

List all surgeries and what year:

-Sleep History-

Do you get restorative/refreshing sleep?
Do your legs feel "restless or jittery" in the evening?
Do you grind your teeth at night?
Does your bed partner say you snore a lot?
Does your bed partner say you kick your legs while asleep?
Do you have acid reflux at night?
Do you sometimes stop breathing when you snore?
Do you ever awaken gagging or fighting for air?

Do you usually awaken with a headache?
Can you easily fall asleep in the afternoon?
Do you sleep walk?
How many hours do you usually sleep?
How many times do you awaken in an average night?
In an *average month* how many mornings do you *wake up feeling refreshed?*
When did you *last* get restorative night's sleep?
_____ years ago . . . or _____ months ago . . . or _____ days ago

-Work Environment-

Describe any significant job stressors:

Describe problems causing loss of efficiency:

Any other major restrictions? (Explain):

-Trauma-

Please list all serious accidents and injuries:

-Stressors-

Please rate your stress levels in relation to the following areas (*no stress, intermittent stress, persistent stress,* or *overwhelming stress*):
Marriage:
Work:
Parents:
Children:
Coworkers:
Financial:
Health:
Other:

-Activity Level-

Please rate according to your *current* level of ability (*often do, sometimes do, never do, couldn't do*):
Read a newspaper:
Shop in a supermarket:
Volunteer your time:
Walk two blocks:
Read a novel:
Do a crossword puzzle:

Clean your house:

Socialize with friends:

Cut your toenails:

Climb two flights of stairs:

Water an indoor plant:

Blow dry your hair:

Walk two miles:

What is the *major* cause for impaired function? (*Circle one*):

Weakness	Restricted motion	Poor vision
Stiffness	Poor concentration	Lack of energy
Immediate pain	Poor balance	Poor motivation
Postexertional pain	Postexertional fatigue	Impaired sensation
Poor coordination	Poor memory	Too much stress
Other reason:		

-Emotional Problems Checklist-

1. Have you been feeling down, depressed, or hopeless in the past month?
2. Are you bothered by little interest or pleasure in doing things?
3. Has your appetite changed (eating more or eating less)?
4. Has your sleep been disturbed (insomnia or oversleeping)?
5. Do you feel worthless or guilty?
6. Do you have sudden or unexpected bouts of anxiety or nervousness?
7. Do you often feel tense, worried, or stressed?
8. Do you have acute onset of symptoms such as palpitations, shortness of breath, or trembling?
9. Do you worry about a lot of different things?
10. Do you avoid places or situations because of anxiety or worry?
11. Do you have recurrent, persistent, or unwanted thoughts or do repetitive behaviors?
12. Have you been through any significantly stressful periods in the past six months?
13. In your lifetime, have you faced any potentially life-threatening events, such as natural disaster, serious accident, physical or sexual assault, military combat, or child abuse?
14. Since you experienced any of these stressors, have you been easily startled? Angry or irritable?
    Emotionally numb or detached from your feelings?
    Prone to physical reactions when reminded of the event?
15. Do you drink alcohol?
16. Do you use prescription medicines or street drugs to relax, calm your nerves, or get high?

17. Have you ever made an effort to cut down on your drinking or drug use?
18. Have you ever been annoyed by people who criticize your drinking or drug use?
19. Do you ever feel guilty about your drinking or drug use?
20. Do you ever drink or use drugs to steady your nerves, get rid of a hangover, or relieve withdrawal symptoms?
21. Do you feel that your eating is out of control?

-Hormonal Issues (Female Patients)-

Have you gone through menopause?   age:
Have you had a total hysterectomy?   age:
Have you had a partial hysterectomy?   age:
Are you perimenopausal
(i.e., still menstruating but having hot flashes)?
Are you taking Estrogens
(e.g., Premarin, Ogen, Estrace, skin patch, etc)?
Are you taking Progestins (e.g., Provera)?
Are you taking birth control pills?

-Unpleasant Leg Sensations-

Do you have an unpleasant, restless feeling in your legs?
If yes, please answer the following questions:
1. Please grade these feelings in the legs as _____ mild _____ moderate _____ severe
2. When do you get these unpleasant feelings? (Check as appropriate):
    _____ in bed at night
    _____ during or after prolonged sitting (such as watching a movie or riding in a car)
    _____ other times (describe_____)
3. Do you have an urge to move your legs during these unpleasant feelings?
4. Are the unpleasant feelings relieved by movements?
5. Do you have any other kinds of feelings in your leg besides "unpleasant and restless"?
    > If yes, circle as appropriate:
    > feeling of insects crawling
    > feeling of worms writhing
    > tingling or numbness
    > pins and needles

-Past Investigations-

Have you had any of the following special investigations? (*Please circle*):

Bone or joint X-rays	Myelogram	Electrocardiogram (ECG)
Radioactive joint scan	Sleep study (polysomnogram)	Echocardiogram (ECHO)
MRI or CT of brain	Mammogram	Laparoscopy
MRI or CT of spine	Electro-encephalogram (EEG)	Arthroscopy
MRI of a joint	Electrical nerve tests (EMG or NCV)	Swallowing studies
Muscle biopsy	Lung function tests (spirometry)	HIV testing
Lymph gland biopsy	CT or MRI of parotid gland	Skin biopsy
Salivary gland biopsy	CT or MRI of chest or abdomen	Ophthalmologic examination
Lumbar puncture	Osteoporosis testing	Angiogram
Balance studies	Abdominal ultrasound	Exploratory surgery
Bladder studies	Schirmer's testing (for dry eyes)	Upper or lower G.I. (endoscopy)
Hearing tests (audiometry)	Visual or auditory evoked potentials	Psychological testing

Any other special studies? (*explain*):

Have you had blood tests within last year?

Have you had a chest X-ray within last year?

Appendix C

Essential Exercises for Fibromyalgia

T he following is a series of essential exercise recommendations for the fibromyalgia
patient written by co-author Janice H. Hoffman, Certified Clinical Exercise
Specialist.

The areas of the body most affected by FM include the abdomen and low back
muscles, chest wall and upper back muscles, front and back thigh muscles, and
lower leg calf muscles. Some of these areas need to be loosened with flexibility
work and others require strengthening to help reduce unnecessary pain and
fatigue in fibromyalgia.

It is common for anyone who sits frequently, either in their work or because of
illness, to need more flexibility in the low back, chest wall, and thighs. When the
human body is seated for long periods, the shoulders tend to slump forward, which
shortens and tightens the chest wall muscles. At the same time, long periods of
sitting cause low back muscles and front and back thigh muscles to grow short and
tight. Meanwhile, prolonged rest keeps calf muscles in a shortened state.

Conversely, as the chest wall tightens the upper back muscles grow weak and
stay in a lengthened position. This creates poor support for the neck and can lead
to headaches as well as upper back pain. And when abdominals grow weak from
disuse, the entire musculature of the lower trunk can lose its girdle-like, stabilizing purpose.

All these postural changes can be corrected with exercises designed to
stretch tight areas and strengthen weak muscles. Effectively strengthening muscles is different for those with FM, since numerous repetitions and long postural

holds can easily bring on a flare. Further, some stretches require working through discomfort at first, when muscles have become very tight. When stretching for flexibility, the length of time a stretch is held and subtle shifts in position can greatly affect how a stretch feels, how challenging it becomes, and whether it is safe.

GENERAL GUIDELINES FOR THE EXERCISES THAT FOLLOW

- Do not exercise cold muscles. Perform five-plus minutes of light rhythmic activity to lubricate joints and warm muscles first. If experiencing a flare, warm the muscles by taking a warm shower before beginning exercise.
- Gently move into the flexibility positions.
- Never tug, bounce, or go beyond a feeling of easy stretching when performing flexibility work.
- Consciously take nice, relaxing inhales and exhales while stretching.
- Add frequent pauses during all strength exercise repetitions.
- Allow a forty-eight-hour rest period between strength work sessions.

FLEXIBILITY

Low Back Flexibility

The low back muscles work in conjunction with the abdominal muscles as stabilizers for the lower torso and pelvis. Prolonged sitting can compress spinal discs and eventually shorten the low back musculature. Elongating these muscles can ease back pain and help them work more effectively in partnership with the abdominals.

Seated Version:

1. Sit tall on a stability ball or sit toward the backrest in a sturdy chair.
2. Gradually lean forward, moving hands down past the knees.
3. Allow the torso and head to relax into gravity's pull.
4. Hold for about ten seconds.

Floor Version:

1. Start face up on a mat or on soft flooring.
2. Bring the thighs toward the chest.
3. Gently press the low back into the floor to lengthen the low back muscles.
4. Hold for about ten seconds.

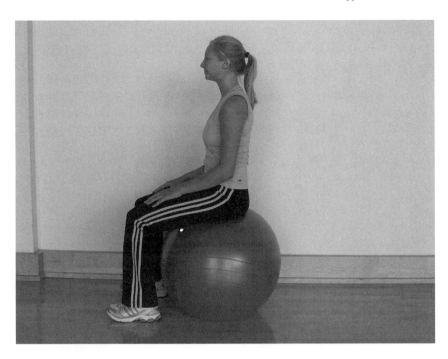

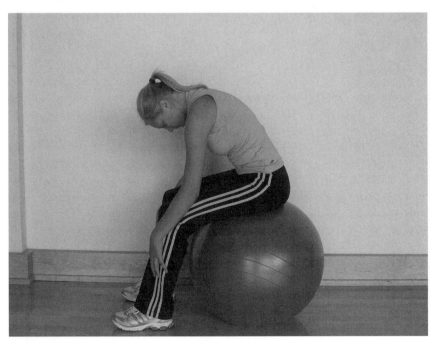

Stability ball exercise for low back flexibility.

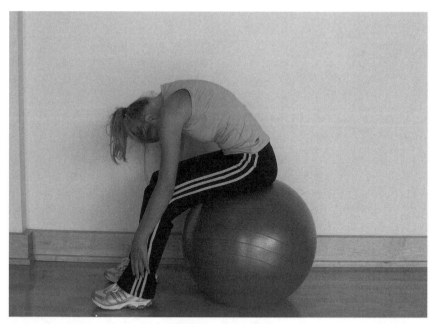

Stability ball exercise for low back flexibility (*continued*).

Where This Stretch Should Be Felt

This stretch will be felt deep in the low back as the torso moves toward the thighs.

How to Do This Stretch Safely

When seated, place hands on thighs for support and slowly walk them down and back up.

Making the Stretch Easier

If seated, do not lean forward as far as pictured.
If face up on the floor, lift just one leg at a time.
Hold the stretch for under ten seconds.

Making the Stretch More Challenging

If seated, move the knees farther apart and bend further toward the floor.
If face up on the floor, move the knees farther apart and lift the tailbone up off the floor.
Hold the stretch for up to twenty seconds.

Chest Wall Flexibility

FM tender-point pain across the upper body can lead to shoulders protectively rolled in, creating tight chest muscles. This stretch is very helpful when done consistently, allowing the shoulders, over time, to move backward into good alignment.

Seated Version:

1. Hold the elbows at shoulder height or slightly below, with fingers near the ears.
2. Continue looking straight ahead and begin to move the elbows from the center toward each side wall.
3. Gently pull the elbows toward the back.
4. Hold for ten seconds.

Standing Version:

1. Stand sideways to a doorway or wall.
2. Raise one arm to shoulder height, or slightly below.
3. Hold onto the doorframe or touch the wall with the extended arm.
4. Slowly turn the body away from the wall.
5. Repeat with the other arm.
6. Hold each side for ten seconds.

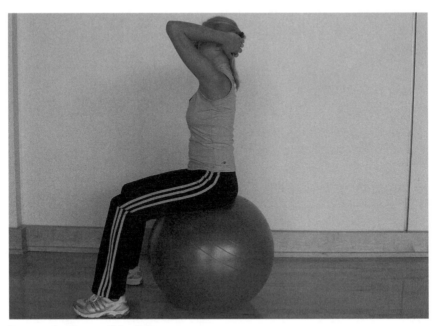

Exercise for chest wall flexibility.

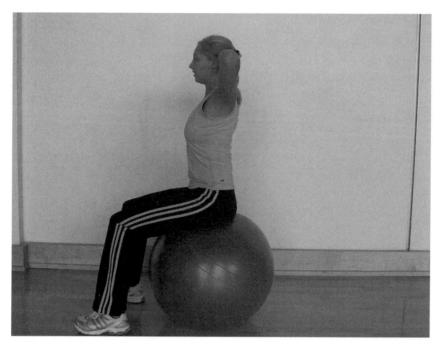

Exercise for chest wall flexibility (*continued*).

Where This Stretch Should Be Felt

This stretch occurs in the front of the upper torso and extends from the breastbone toward the shoulders and upper arms.

How to Do This Stretch Safely

Do not arch the lower back.
Look straight ahead throughout the stretch.
Keep the elbows slightly bent.

Making the Stretch Easier

Hold the arms below shoulder height without touching the head and open the arms to the side and backward.
Hold the stretch for under ten seconds.

Making the Stretch More Challenging

Increase the degree at which the elbows move backward.
Hold the stretch for up to twenty seconds.

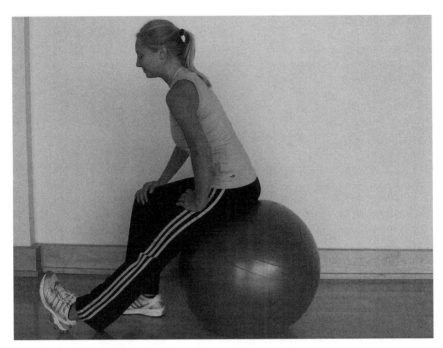

Exercise for thigh flexibility.

Back of Thigh Flexibility

The hamstring muscles are located in the back of the upper thigh. They work together with the major muscles in the front of the thigh to move the hip and the knees. Many people, not just those with FM, have tight hamstring muscles from extended sitting. Being able to move a straightened leg to a 90-degree angle from the torso is considered normal hamstring flexibility.

Seated Version:

1. Sit squarely on the stability ball, or sit away from the chair back.
2. Extend one leg straight out, with the heel touching the floor.
3. Lean forward from the hips.
4. Keep the back very flat "like a table top."
5. Hold for about ten seconds.
6. Repeat with the other leg.

Floor Version:

1. Lie on the floor face up with knees bent and feet on the floor.
2. Lift one leg, straightening the knee.

3. Hold for about ten seconds.
4. Repeat with the other leg.

Where This Stretch Should Be Felt

This stretch centers along the back of the thigh from the buttocks to the knee. Some continuing pull may be felt down into the calf region, especially if the foot is flexed during the stretch.

How to Do This Stretch Safely

If face up on the floor, keep the shoulder blades on the floor.
If face up on the floor, do not lift the head up.
If seated, do not press on the extended leg with the hands.

Making the Stretch Easier

Seated: While keeping the back straight, do not bend forward very far.
On the floor: Use a stretch strap or long towel at the underside of the foot as an arm "extension."
Hold the stretch for under ten seconds.

Making the Stretch More Challenging

Decrease the position angle between torso and body to less than 90 degrees.
Hold the stretch for up to twenty seconds.

Hip Flexibility

The large muscles between the torso and legs are among the most powerful in the body. Poor mobility and tightness in these muscles can cause problems to occur from the low back to the knees.

Seated Version:

1. Sit sideways on a chair or stability ball with the legs in a lunge position.
2. Tilt the tailbone forward and up, toward the ceiling.
3. Hold about ten seconds.
4. Repeat facing the other direction with the other leg.

Standing Version:

1. Stand tall with the legs in a lunge position.
2. Bend and lower the front and back knees, sinking slightly toward the floor.

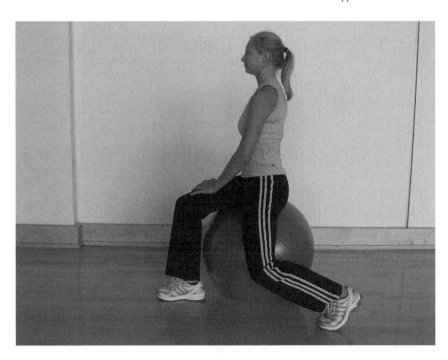

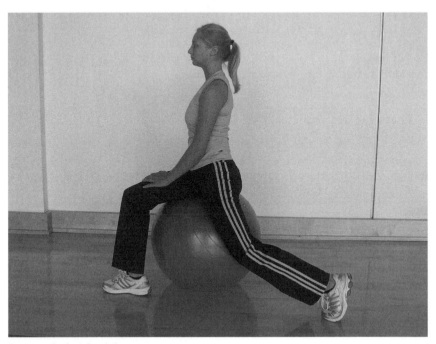

Exercise for hip flexibility.

3. Tilt the tailbone forward and up, toward the ceiling.
4. Hold about ten seconds.
5. Change the lunge position to the other leg and repeat steps 2 through 4.

Where This Stretch Should Be Felt

This stretch will pull at the junction between the front of the torso and thigh on the back leg.

How to Do This Stretch Safely

Don't allow the low back to arch into a curve.

If standing, keep the front knee from moving over and ahead of the toes.

When seated on a stability ball, if balance is an issue, work near a wall or hold onto the side of the ball with both hands.

Making the Stretch Easier

Tilt the pelvis forward less.

Hold the stretch for under ten seconds.

Making the Stretch More Challenging

Tilt the pelvis further forward and up, to deepen the pull.

Hold the stretch for up to twenty seconds.

Lower Leg and Foot Flexibility

Tight muscles in the calves and the soles of the feet can occur during extended inactivity. Stretching the back of the lower legs, around the ankle joints, and keeping the fascia in the soles of the feet lengthened can prevent leg cramping and ease the pain of plantar fasciitis.

Floor Version:

1. Stand with feet about hip width apart.
2. Place one foot forward and one foot back, keeping toes directed straight ahead.
3. Bend the front knee and lean forward, keeping the back heel pressed down.
4. Hold about ten seconds.
5. Repeat with the other leg.

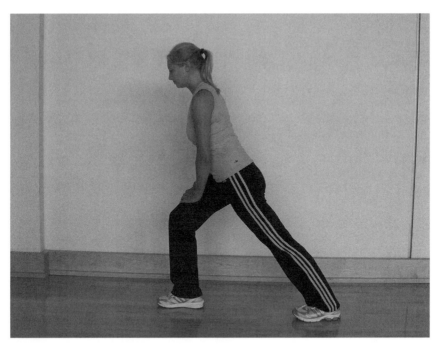

Exercise for lower-leg and foot flexibility.

Where This Stretch Should Be Felt

In the soles of the feet and the calves, including a sense of pull extending up toward the knee joint.

How to Do This Stretch Safely

Place a hand on the thigh for good back support.
Do not press on the knee joint.
To help prevent neck strain, keep the entire body on a diagonal.

Making the Stretch Easier

Move the back leg closer toward the body's centerline.
Hold the stretch for under ten seconds.

Making the Stretch More Challenging

Move the back leg farther back, away from the body's centerline.
Hold the stretch for up to twenty seconds.

STRENGTH WORK

Abdominal Wall Strengthening

The abdominal muscles are important for spinal stability and injury prevention, especially for the low back. The abdominal muscles work mainly as stabilizing postural muscles. They are designed to stay active for long periods of time. When weakened, imbalances can occur between the coordinating muscles of the low back.

Floor Version:

1. Lie face up the floor with knees bent and hands by hips.
2. Lift one leg up until it is perpendicular with the floor.
3. Then slowly release the leg back down to the floor.
4. Repeat with the other leg.
5. Perform from five to ten repetitions with each leg.

Where This Work Should Be Felt

The goal of the exercise is to use the abdominal muscles to lift the legs, not the back muscles. The back muscles should stay relaxed.

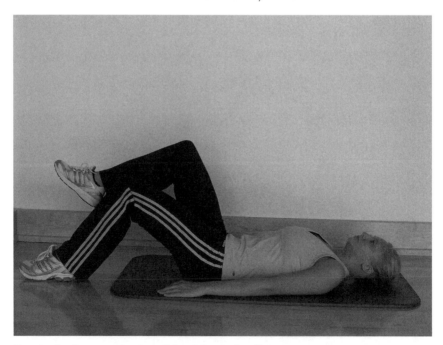

Exercise for the strengthening of the abdominal wall.

How to Perform This Work Safely

- Persons with FM need to keep the exercise work repetitions (the cycle from one beginning movement to the end movement before repeating) low. Perform a maximum of ten repetitions before resting for at least thirty seconds.
- Abdominal muscles need to be worked in a slow fashion, without jerking or using momentum to start the movement.
- Although abdominal muscles need to be tight throughout the movement, remember to breathe.

Making This Work Easier

To reduce any strain on the lower back and to help use abdominal muscles to lift legs, place a folded towel or a yoga wedge under buttocks.

Perform fewer repetitions.

Making This Work More Challenging

Change to a toe tap rather than placing the whole foot down.

Lift and lower both legs together.

Gradually add more repetitions.

Upper Back Strengthening

Persons with FM have a series of tender points that run along the upper back muscles, making this a tender area to move. This often results in muscle inactivity. However, the muscles need to be kept strong since weak upper back muscles can result in more neck, upper back, and shoulder pain.

Stability Ball Version:

1. Begin by kneeling in front of a stability ball on a padded surface.
2. Place hands behind head, elbows pointing to the floor.
3. Gradually lift the torso away from the stability ball using the shoulder blade area to do the work.
4. Gently squeeze the shoulder blades together and lift the elbows to feel the work moving into the back of the shoulders.
5. Lower slowly.
6. Perform five to ten repetitions.

Where This Work Should Be Felt

Working the upper back should result in a sense of fatigue between the shoulder blades and possibly in the back shoulder muscles. Additionally, if the chest

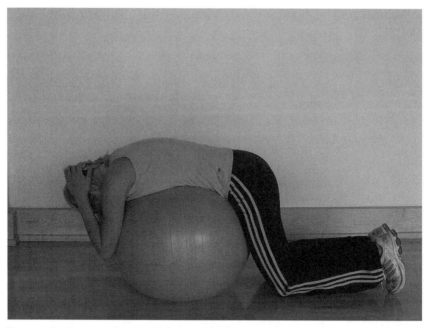

Exercise for the strengthening of the upper back.

muscles are very tight, the exerciser may feel a pulling sensation at that location. Avoid allowing the abdominals to pull the body upward.

How to Do This Work Safely

- Persons with FM need to keep the exercise work repetitions (the cycle from one beginning movement to the end movement before repeating) low. Perform a maximum of ten repetitions before resting for at least thirty seconds.
- Work in a rhythmic fashion, going slow enough that there is no momentum being used to take the work away from the affected muscles.
- Keep the neck in line with the spine for the entire movement by keeping eyes on the floor.
- Remember to breathe.

Making This Work Easier

Perform fewer repetitions.

Making This Work More Challenging

Gradually increase the repetitions.

Appendix D

Dietary Recommendations for Fibromyalgia Patients

The following is a series of practical dietary recommendations for the fibromyalgia patient written by Katie Holton, MPH.

It is no surprise that many people find it challenging these days to know how to eat healthy, much less how to lose weight. We are bombarded with conflicting information that we are left to wade through on our own. This article will give you some solid strategies that you can use no matter if your quest is to lose weight or just to improve your diet in the hopes of improving your fibromyalgia symptoms.

1. "Diet" just means "what you eat." There are plenty of diet fads being advertised these days that tell people how to drastically change their diets if they want to look like a model. If you go "on" a diet to lose weight, what do you expect to happen when you go "off" the diet? To optimize health and to lose weight, you really need to alter your thinking toward a gradual change of eating habits for the long-term.

2. The 90 percent–10 percent rule. Think about eating optimally 90 percent of the time, and that 10 percent of the time you can be a little more lax. Trying to lose weight is not like recovering from alcoholism. You cannot fall off the wagon! But what you do the majority of the time *will* drive your success or impede your progress.

3. Focus on balance. The fad weight-loss diets that tell you to remove one of the macronutrients (namely carbohydrates or fat) are easier to follow, not from an eating standpoint, but just by the simple fact that it is easy to tell if something is "in" or "out." Unfortunately, your body needs all three macronutrients, and removing or increasing one of them will always result in an imbalance that puts your body at risk. Not all carbs, proteins, or fats are created equal, so the choices you make in each area matter. For carbohydrates, focus first on vegetables, whole fruit (not juice), and beans which are most nutrient dense. Then choose small amounts of whole-grain products, trying to limit/remove all foods containing refined grains like white flour and sugar. For fat, avoid trans fats, which are found in processed foods, and limit your intake of saturated fats, which are found in animal fat, such as lard, butter, cheese, whole milk, ice cream, and meat. Make low-fat choices for dairy and buy the leanest cuts of meat you can find. Increasing omega-3 fatty acids has been shown to benefit health greatly. So increase your consumption of cold-water fish like wild (not farm-raised) salmon, walnuts, grain products with ground flax seed, and eggs which are labeled higher in omega-3s. High-quality, nutrient-dense foods should be your goal.

4. Avoid additives. This point is very important! A quick and easy rule of thumb is to look at all ingredient lists, and if they are long and contain chemical names that are difficult to understand, don't eat it! There are many chemicals added to our food: preservatives, artificial colors and flavors, and flavor enhancers. These all could have long-term effects on health, and some will affect both cravings toward a food item and how you feel after eating them. Search for foods with very few ingredients that you can read without a PhD. Tip: Be wary of sauces and mixed spices. Try using simple vinaigrettes for your salad as opposed to processed dressings like ranch or Caesar.

5. Avoid artificial sweeteners. Our bodies adapt to exposures. If a person eats sugar on a daily basis, they will find themselves craving sugar on subsequent days. Artificial sweeteners are actually much sweeter than sugar and make the body crave sweetness even more than sugar. This increases cravings, which in turn hampers weight loss. By removing all artificial sweeteners from the diet and by limiting your intake of sugar (especially high-fructose corn syrup), you can actually increase your body's ability to taste sweetness in healthy foods, like vegetables and fruit. Watch out for gum, breath mints, and medications which all can be hidden sources of artificial sweeteners. You can find safe versions of these at your local health food store, but still be careful to read labels as not all items at the health food store are safe.

6. Keep a diary. Don't worry; you don't have to count calories! Simply keeping track of what you eat, when you eat it, and how you feel in the hours afterward can help you greatly in identifying patterns in your eating and reactions to certain foods. This is especially important for those with fibromyalgia, whether weight loss is a desired goal or not. This habit will help you be more aware of food-induced sensations (GI disturbance, fatigue, cravings, etc.) and will help reinforce how great you feel when eating whole, unprocessed foods like vegetables and fruits. When eating out, add the name of the restaurant and meal eaten in your diary to help you find places that aid you in your healthy eating.

7. Don't increase carbohydrate intake to increase energy levels. Everyone knows that carbs are the body's energy source, so many mistakenly think that increasing the amount of carbs they eat will give them more energy and ease the fatigue associated with fibromyalgia. This can lead to spikes in blood sugar that cause a corresponding "low" blood sugar period. In a state of hypoglycemia (low blood sugar) the body feels the need to regulate itself back to "normal." You may feel shaky and weak, have foggy thinking, and will crave simple sugars. If items with simple sugars are eaten, it can actually re-spike the blood sugar, with temporary relief, but then the same pattern continues. Instead, think of eating foods together in a balanced manner. Some examples of this would be eating an apple with natural peanut butter (short list of ingredients would be peanuts and salt), soybeans (which are naturally balanced), or eggs and fruit for breakfast. Think of aiming for a little protein, fat, and carbs (preferably high in fiber) at every meal and snack. This will help slow the rise in blood sugar and prevent the spikes and dips. The two hardest times of day for most people are breakfast and snacks. Many breakfast foods in the United States tend to be very high in simple sugars (cereals, pancakes, pastries, etc.) and should be avoided. Better choices are things like slow-cooking oatmeal with milk or plain yogurt with frozen berries and wheat germ added.

8. Careful with caffeine. It is common to want to try to self medicate with caffeine in order to attempt to improve fatigue symptoms. Be cautious of doing so, as it can lead you into a vicious cycle of poor sleep habits. If a person is feeling fatigued in the afternoon or evening and then has caffeine, it can keep the person from entering their deep sleep at night, which then results in increased tiredness (and need for sleep) the next day. This cycle can be perpetuated over time with gradual decreases in function caused by inadequate sleep. This can increase fibromyalgia symptoms and should be avoided.

9. Special note about medications. Many fibromyalgia medications cause gastrointestinal symptoms. Pay special attention to how you feel after taking medications and note effects on appetite and GI function. Some symptoms may be caused by your medication and may be alleviated with a change in your prescription. If you feel like you are having difficulty eating properly, you may also be deficient in many nutrients that your body needs on a daily basis, which inhibits healing, sleep, and daily function. If dietary changes result in improvements in your symptoms, you may be able to discuss weaning off medications with your health care provider.

Overall, remember that nothing influences your health as much as diet. And most important, it is something that is completely under your control. Take back your health using the approaches outlined earlier. Eating healthy is about making slow, steady changes in the right direction, not about suddenly starting a new "diet" that won't be continued for the long run. Give yourself small goals like replacing all beverages during the day with water. Then add to this the next week with another small goal. And then reward yourself with a new outfit or a special trip to celebrate your weight loss or how great you feel!

SAMPLE BREAKFAST

Slow-cooking oatmeal (takes five minutes in the microwave) with milk or water

Vanilla yogurt (try to find a brand with very few ingredients like milk, sugar, vanilla, and bacteria—avoid gelatin, artificial sweeteners, and artificial colors)

Apples—chopped

Cinnamon (to taste)

Cook oatmeal for five minutes in a microwave with either milk or water. Add some vanilla yogurt (for sweetness), cinnamon, and chopped up apples. Stir and serve.

For an Even Quicker Breakfast:

Heat up a 1/2 cup of frozen berries in the microwave long enough for a juice to form.

Then add to vanilla (or plain) yogurt and stir until color changes.

Sprinkle top with wheat germ and a little granola cereal.

Higher Protein Breakfast:

Sauté chopped green pepper, onion, and garlic with olive or canola oil in a frying pan.

Add two eggs and scramble

Salt and pepper to taste

Fresh sliced fruit

Serve with a slice of toast (try to find a nutty, grainy bread with no additives) with a tablespoon of honey or jam.

SAMPLE LUNCH

Tuna Sandwich:

Whole-grain bread with no additives

Tuna packed in water (try to find one *without* broth on the ingredient list)

Mayonnaise (canola oil mayo or flax oil mayo are good choices)

Celery, onion

Salt and pepper to taste

Fresh, raw veggies like cut-up carrots (try to have veggies at lunch and dinner or as snacks)

Fresh fruit (apple, orange, etc.)

Note: Deli meat is high in additives and is better purchased from health food store delis. Try finding a healthier alternative to deli meat you like and creating sandwiches with whole-grain (low additive) bread, mayo/mustard, lettuce, tomato, and onion.

Snacking through lunch can be good for you if you choose healthy items. Always start with fresh veggies and fruit. You can add protein by dipping apple slices in peanut butter or having hard-boiled eggs. Nuts (raw or with salt) are a good choice to balance blood sugar as well. And *avoid* canned soups for lunch and dinner due to additive content.

Salad: Try making a salad with a mix of greens. Add chopped veggies and sliced hard-boiled egg (or leftover chicken) for protein. Find a dressing with few ingredients like oil, vinegar, and whole spices.

SAMPLE DINNER

Keep dinner balanced with protein, carbohydrates, and fat.

Try to pick lean cuts of meat with no additives, sauces, or marinades.

Always have vegetables at dinnertime.

If you include starchy foods, keep portions small and choose healthy carbs like:

Brown or wild rice, small baked potato (eat the skin!), or whole-wheat pasta.

Make your own marinades and add only whole spices!

Sit with friends and family and enjoy the social aspects of eating.

Chicken Fajitas

Boneless, skinless chicken—sliced

Marinade: 1/4 c. canola oil, 1/4 c. red wine vinegar, 1 T. Oregano, 1 tsp. chili powder, 1 tsp. garlic powder (or fresh crushed garlic), 1 tsp. salt, 1/4 tsp. pepper

Sliced green and red peppers

Sliced onion

Mix marinade together with sliced chicken, peppers, and onion. Marinate chicken mix for four to twenty-four hours and then either pan fry or place in slow cooker. Serve with whole-wheat Mexican-brand tortillas (should have very few ingredients) or corn tortillas and mild or medium cheddar cheese. Cooked fajita mix is wonderful over a salad, too, and dressing is not normally needed.

Appendix E

Conversations between a Counselor and a Client with Fibromyalgia

The following example of a counseling session was written by Rebecca Ross RN, PhD, Psychiatric Mental Health Nurse Practitioner:

The purpose of this appendix is to depict conversations between a counselor and a patient with fibromyalgia (FM). The theme of the interaction is "The 'New Normal': Thriving in the Here and Now!" Many people who are newly diagnosed with a chronic illness such as FM struggle with the forced changes in their lives. Fibromyalgia-related changes occur in many spheres of life:

- *Physical ability*
- *Energy level*
- *Cognitive ability*
- *Social function*
- *Financial stability*
- *Role expectations (spouse, parent, employee, etc).*

These core areas are essential to address in order to regain balance in all spheres of life. These changes are not only difficult for people with FM but also for their family, friends, and coworkers. Here is an excerpt from a typical counseling session.

Counselor

It is important to identify your "New Normal," as your predisease state and level of functioning is very different from your current functioning with FM.

No one wants to have a chronic illness and the role changes that inevitably follow. However, if one is to attain maximal health, the new normal needs to be communicated with others. People who have been used to your role of wife, caregiver, friend, sister, parent, etc. and have relied on your assistance will not be able to let go of their expectations as easily as one might think. Therefore, it is important for *you* to identify what you can and cannot do so you do not worsen your condition. You need to communicate your new limitations in an effective, healthy conversation. What is most difficult for you right now?

Client

I can't get my husband to understand that he needs to take a more active role with the children. For example, last night I asked him to bathe the kids. He replied that he "needed to 'wind down' from work." He reminded me that when we got married, we decided that I would stay home and take care of the kids and he would work outside of the home. Now I feel guilty that I can't do "my job" and I am letting him down. It isn't fair to put the entire burden on him, but I can't bathe the kids anymore due to my pain.

Counselor

First, let me ask you, "if the situations were reversed, would you be mad or disappointed with your husband, or would you understand that changes were required because of his disease"? Most people answer that "of course they would understand and that they would take care of what needed to be done and not begrudge needed changes. Having said that, role re-negotiation really is an important step in reestablishing a healthy balance within the family. For instance, if your pain or fatigue limits you from completing the full one-hour bath time ritual, split the task into less physical and most physical dimensions. Ask your husband to do those things are most painful or fatiguing to you. For example, you might run the bath water and set out pajamas while he actually oversees the bathing. Do you think that would work for both of you?

Client

Yes, I will try that.

Counselor

What else is challenging for you?

Client

Our big family meal is usually dinner. But now I am too tired to shop, cook, and clean the kitchen at night.

Counselor

Pacing activities and reassigning duties can be very helpful. For instance, if you can write the shopping list for the week, perhaps he can shop. Also, some tasks could be done earlier in the day, such as setting the table or preparing a side dish or preparing the kitchen for cooking. Alternatively, the main purpose of family dinner is to spend time together communicating. Many families adopt easier dinner menus such as soup, sandwiches, or even breakfast items. Another option may be healthy restaurant take-out. Would any of these options work for you?

Client

I think he would be willing to stop by a restaurant for take-out food on his way home from work if I ordered the meal. Another problem lately is my memory. I have a hard time remembering our family schedule, such as medical and dental appointments and play dates for the kids.

Counselor

Many people complain of "fibro-fog" which affects people's ability to multitask and remember things without writing them down. One suggestion is to get a large wall calendar and put it in a central location so that everyone in the family can see it often. Family planner organizational systems are available with stickers reminding people of key events. Don't be hesitant to make lists or use sticky notes. Another one of my clients uses a "launching pad" system. She puts everything that needs to be taken to school or appointments in a basket next to the front door. Then she sees them as she is leaving and picks them up. She also has a basket next to her couch for the household bills/paperwork. Then she can sit down and rest while she attends to these items. How are you doing with social activities?

Client

I am too tired most of the time. When I do schedule something with my friends or extended family, I often have to cancel at the last minute. It is difficult for people to understand since I look healthy. My friends rarely call anymore. My husband and I used to go out to dinner and a movie once a week, but I'm too tired to arrange childcare and endure four hours away from home.

Counselor

This is very hard as FM is an invisible illness; people do not understand your limitations because you don't look sick. There are many strategies you can use to schedule pleasant activities and self-care. These might include: (1) ask your friends to continue to include you in activities, but drive your own car so you can leave at your discretion, (2) continue "date night" with your husband, but ask him to schedule the babysitting and consider one activity only, such as dinner or a movie, and (3) schedule activities during your best time of day (e.g., brunch instead of dinner).

Client

These are great ideas. I can do some of them, but it is increasingly difficult to go out due to my rising medical bills. I feel guilty spending money on myself, especially since my medical bills have become a financial burden.

Counselor

There are many strategies to remain socially active while minimizing costs. Some people meet at the park and enjoy a sandwich made at home rather than going out to a restaurant. Others meet for coffee rather than a full meal. Focus on enjoying the time together rather than the actual food.

Client

My family is accustomed to me doing a lot for them. I used to be able to take care of the house, meals, kids, yard, and help with our aging parents. Now I'm too tired or in too much pain to take care of anyone other than myself or my kids. My husband rarely complains, but I can tell that he misses the way things used to be. Frankly, I miss being able to help everyone and that makes me feel guilty and worthless.

Counselor

We call what you are describing "role strain." Basically, you have had to change all your roles, and you need to let go of what you used to be able to do. Setting priorities is very helpful. Make a list of the top five priorities for the day and adapt your expectations to how you feel that day. Discuss these priorities with your family and ask what tasks are most important to them. You may be surprised by their answers. For example, they may not be as concerned about a clean house as they are spending time watching a home movie with you.

Glossary

acellular Unable to grow through cell division.

acetaminophen A common over-the-counter medication used for the relief of fever, headaches, and minor aches and pains. This class of drugs are called analgesics (pain relievers) and antipyretics (fever reducers).

ACh (acetylcholine) One of many neurotransmitters in the ANS and the only neurotransmitter used in the somatic nervous system.

ACR (American College of Rheumatology) The official organization for health-care professionals who treat arthritis and other rheumatic diseases.

acupuncture points Areas of the body thought by many practitioners to stimulate the body's natural energy and promote healing when stimulated by insertion of small needles.

ADD (Attention Deficit Disorder) A neurobehavioral disorder characterized by a persistent impulsiveness and inattention, and sometimes including hyperactivity (ADHD).

adrenaline See epinephrine

allodynia Pain from stimuli that are not normally painful. The term includes pain that occurs in another area than in the one stimulated.

allopathic A term commonly used to indicate traditional or Western medicine.

alpha-2 delta receptor blockers Medications like gabapentin and pregabalin that affect voltage-regulated calcium channels in the central nervous system, slowing the release of excitatory neurotransmitters.

amygdala Considered by many as the brain's primitive seat of emotions.

ANA test (antinuclear antibody test) A laboratory blood test that diagnoses inflammatory diseases. It measures the pattern and amount of autoantibody that might attack tissues as if they were foreign material.

analgesics A drug or medicine given to reduce pain without resulting in loss of consciousness. Analgesics are sometimes referred to as painkiller medications. There are many different types of analgesic medications available in both prescription and over-the-counter preparations.

anaphylactic reaction A potentially life-threatening allergic reaction that may occur after ingestion, skin contact, or injection of an allergen or, in some cases, inhalation of an allergen.

anemia Anemia is the most common disorder of the blood. The three main causes of anemia include excessive blood loss, excessive blood cell destruction, or poor red blood cell production.

anesthesia Having sensation, especially pain, blocked or temporarily taken away. General anesthesia is the common term for the loss of consciousness induced by drugs given before and during surgery.

ANS (Autonomic Nervous System) The portion of the nervous system that controls the function of organ systems for the body.

anti-emetic A drug that is effective against vomiting and nausea. Anti-emetics are typically used to treat motion sickness and the side effects of opioid analgesics, chemotherapy, or drugs used during general anesthesia.

antibiotics A chemotherapeutic agent with activity against microorganisms such as bacteria.

apnea A term for the lack of movement in the breathing muscles while the volume of air in the lungs remains unchanged. Apnea can be voluntary (breath-holding), drug-induced, or can occur as a consequence of neurological disease or trauma.

arginine An amino acid classified as conditionally essential, depending on the developmental stage and health status of the individual.

articular rheumatism A type of rheumatic disease involving joint deformity.

Attention Deficit Disorder See ADD

autoimmune disease An overactive immune response of the body against substances and tissues normally present in the body.

Autonomic Nervous System See ANS

Axis II disorders One of five psychiatric classifications, Axis II disorders include the following: paranoid personality disorder, schizoid personality disorder, borderline personality disorder, antisocial personality disorder, narcissistic personality disorder, histrionic personality disorder, avoidant personality disorder, dependent personality disorder, obsessive-compulsive personality disorder, and mental retardation.

bipolar disorder A mood disorder defined by one or more episodes of abnormally elevated mood called manic episodes. Individuals who experience manic episodes also commonly experience depressive symptoms.

body pain diagram A body drawing patients shade in to help the clinician visualize which areas have hurt for most days of the week over the past three months.

bruxism Grinding one's teeth, especially at night. Associated with TMD. Clenching is separate from bruxism and also worsens TMD and wears teeth unnaturally.

bursitis The inflammation of one or more sacs of synovial fluid in the body.

cardiac Referring to the heart.

Catechol-O-methyl transferase gene See COMT gene

cataplexy A medical condition that affects people who have narcolepsy. Cataplexy is sometimes confused with epilepsy because it produces similar seizures. The term originates from the Greek words *kata* (down) and *plexis* (stroke).

catecholamine Act as modulators in the central nervous system and as hormones in the blood circulation (see epinephrine and norepinephrine). High blood levels of catecholamine are associated with stress.

Celiac Disease (CD) A digestive disorder to which people are genetically predisposed that causes damage to the mucosal surface of the small intestine. It is a result of an immunologically toxic reaction to the ingestion of gluten.

central nervous system See CNS

central sensitization (CS) An imbalance of electrical activity and neurotransmitters that unnaturally excite amino acids in the brain and spinal cord. It is chronic pain that goes untreated and increases in intensity, spreading from an original site to body areas that weren't previously affected, further damaging health and functioning. CS causes heightened awareness of external stimuli, including noise, light, smell, and touch.

cerebral spinal fluid The fluid content that flows over the brain as well as the central canal of the spinal cord. It acts as a cushion and provides basic mechanical and immunological protection inside the skull and spinal vertebrae.

chemokines A family of small cytokines, or proteins, secreted by cells.

Chiari malformation An anatomical problem in which part of the brain stem, the cerebellar tonsils, protrudes downward toward the spinal column.

chronic pain Pain that persists or progresses over a long period of time, generally greater than three months. This is in contrast to acute pain that arises suddenly in response to a specific injury and is usually treatable. Chronic pain persists over time and is often resistant to medical treatments.

co-morbidities Overlapping but separate disorders or symptoms.

CNS (central nervous system) A part of the nervous system that functions to coordinate activity. It consists of the brain in the cranial cavity and the spinal cord in the spinal cavity. Together with the peripheral nervous system it has a fundamental role in the control of behavior.

cognition The process of thought.

COMT gene (Catechol-O-methyl transferase gene) One of several enzymes that degrade dopamine, epinephrine, and norepinephrine, which are catecholamines. The regulation of catecholamine is impaired in a number of medical conditions. Certain medications target COMT and alter its activity by providing better availability of catecholamines.

cortisol A hormone produced by the adrenal cortex. It is usually referred to as the stress hormone because it is involved in the body's response to stress. It increases blood pressure and reduces immune response. Synthetic cortisol is prescribed to treat a variety of illnesses. More recently, cortisol is being researched for its connection with abnormal hormonal levels, clinical depression, psychological stress, and physiological stressors.

Coxsackie Refers to a group of viruses that triggers illness ranging from mild GI distress to serious heart conditions. Symptoms of infection with viruses in the Coxsackie B grouping include fever, headache, sore throat, gastrointestinal distress, as well as chest and muscle pain.

cytokine Protein, peptide, or glycoprotein molecules that, like hormones and neurotransmitters, are used in cellular communication. Cytokines are critical to the development and functioning of immune response although not limited to just the immune system. They are often secreted by immune cells that have encountered a pathogen, thereby activating and recruiting further immune cells to increase the system's response to the pathogen. From the Greek words *cyto* (cell) and *kinos* (movement).

dementia A decline in cognitive function due to damage or disease in the body. From the Latin words *de* (apart) and *mentis* (mind).

diagnostic criteria Combined signs, symptoms, and test results that allow clinicians to diagnose disease.

disequilibrium Loss or lack of stability, dizziness, or vertigo.

disorder A set of symptoms that are clearly connected by objective, reproducible pathophysiologic changes.

dopamine This is a key neurotransmitter that plays a critical role in regulating pain perception and pain relief. It is perhaps best known for its various roles in Parkinson's disease, schizophrenia, and drug addiction.

dorsal horn An area in the back of the spinal cord that receives sensory information from the body including touch, proprioception, and vibration. The needed information is received from receptors of the skin, bones, and joints through sensory neurons.

downregulation A calming of pain perception. An example of downregulation is the cellular decrease in the number of receptors, such as a hormone or neuro-transmitter to a molecule, which in turn reduces the cell's sensitivity to that molecule. An increase of a cellular component is called upregulation.

dry needling The use of a moving, solid needle for therapy, in contrast to the use of a hollow hypodermic needle to inject substances such as saline solution to the same point. Acupuncture is one example of dry needling.

dysautonomia The medical term for autonomic nervous system (ANS) dysfunction.

dyslexia A learning disability involving difficulty with written language, especially reading and spelling. It is separate and distinct from reading difficulties resulting from other causes.

dysmenorrhea A condition characterized by severe and frequent menstrual cramps and pain.

endocrine gland Any of various glands producing hormonal secretions passing directly into the bloodstream. The endocrine glands include thyroid, parathyroid, anterior and posterior pituitary, pancreas, adrenals, pineal, and gonads.

endometriosis A medical condition in women in which endometrial cells are deposited in areas outside the uterine cavity. Symptoms often exacerbate in time with the menstrual cycle. From the Latin words *endo* (inside) and *metra* (womb).

endorphins The body's natural pain killers; also associated with exercise-induced "runners high."

epidemiology The study of factors affecting the health of various populations.

epinephrine A neurotransmitter and stress hormone. It is considered the predominant sympathetic neurotransmitter in the ANS. From the Greek words *epi* (upon) and *nephros* (kidney). It refers to the adrenal gland just above the kidneys where epinephrine is produced.

Epstein-Barr See HHV-4

fibro-fog States of confusion, poor attention and concentration, short-term memory loss, and slowed processing.

fibrositis The former name for fibromyalgia (FM).

flare A period in which disease symptoms reappear or become worse.

FM (fibromyalgia) A disorder characterized by chronic pain, stiffness, and tenderness of muscles, tendons, and joints without detectable inflammation. Sleep disorders are common. FM does not cause body damage or deformity. Undue fatigue plagues the large majority of patients with FM.

fMRI (functional MRI imaging) A technique for visualizing metabolic activity in the brain in "real time." Used in FM during a painful stimulus.

functional brain imaging See fMRI

genetic marker Similar to a blood type, genetic markers are specific tissue types or genes that are passed from parents to their offspring. Some genetic markers are linked to certain rheumatic diseases.

GHDS (growth hormone deficiency syndrome) A medical condition in which the body does not produce enough growth hormone. Growth hormone, also called somatotropin, stimulates growth and cell reproduction.

glucose testing Laboratory tests of blood, serum, or urine commonly used to detect diabetes.

healthy control A person in a clinical trial who has no known diseases, or at least not the disease under study.

heart palpitations Physical sensation of irregularities in the beating of the heart.

heart rate variability Electrical stimulation patterns produced by the autonomic nervous system and recorded on specialized equipment. An objective test of dysautonomia.

Hepatitis C A viral chronic liver infection that is thought to be a trigger for the onset of FM in genetically susceptible persons.

Herpes Lymphotropic Virus See acetylcholine

HGH (human growth hormone) A small polypeptide released by the pituitary gland in the presence of high levels of growth-hormone-releasing hormone and low levels of hypothalamic somatostatin.

HHV-4 (Epstein-Barr) This is one of the world's most common viruses. When it occurs during adolescence, it often causes mononucleosis. There is ongoing debate about the significance or treatment for chronic HHV-4 infection.

HHV-6 (Herpes Lymphotropic Virus) A classification or genus of the herpes virus.

hippocampal complex A part of the forebrain, located in the medial temporal lobe, belonging to the limbic system.

HIV The human immunodeficiency virus, a type of retrovirus that, if left untreated, leads to acquired immunodeficiency syndrome (AIDS).

HPA (hypothalamic-pituitary-adrenal axis) A major part of the neuroendocrine system that controls reactions to stress and regulates many body processes. The hypothalamus and pituitary are part of the brain, whereas the adrenals are above the kidneys.

human growth hormone See HGH

hyperlipidemia Raised or abnormal levels of lipids such as cholesterol or triglycerides in the bloodstream.

hypersomnia Excessive daytime sleepiness, often resulting in falling asleep at dangerous or inappropriate times.

hypothesis Refers to any idea worthy of evaluation but still requiring more work by researchers to confirm or disprove its worth as a theory. A confirmed hypothesis may become part of a theory or occasionally may grow to become a theory itself.

hypothyroidism A disease of the thyroid gland in which inadequate thyroid hormone is produced.

IB (Irritable Bladder) Irritable bladder is a general term for a number of diseases or disorders that provokes the muscles in the bladder to contract involuntarily, resulting in a sudden, urgent, uncontrollable need to urinate (urge incontinence).

IBD (Inflammatory Bowel Disease) An autoimmune disease of the intestines. Symptoms are varied but often include abdominal cramps, diarrhea, bloody stools, and inflammation. Other body organs such as the eyes or joints may also be involved.

IBS (Irritable Bowel Syndrome) A common gastrointestinal disorder involving abnormal gut motility (contractions) or autonomic dysfunction and characterized by abdominal pain, bloating, mucous in stools, and alternating diarrhea and constipation. Symptoms tend to be chronic and wax and wane over the years. Although IBS can cause chronic recurrent discomfort, it does not lead to serious organ problems.

IGF-1 (Insulin-like Growth Factor) A polypeptide secreted mainly by the liver in response to stimulation by growth hormone from the pituitary.

inflammatory bowel disease See IBD

insomnia Difficulty falling asleep, difficulty staying asleep, or early morning waking.

Insulin-like Growth Factor See IGF-1

interstitial cystitis Chronic (long-term) inflammation of the bladder wall.

irritable bowel syndrome See IBS

laboratory markers Biological specimens that can be measured with tests or equipment and that may be used to diagnose illness.

LDL levels A type of lipoprotein with at least five subtypes. Each is thought to be of varying value in cholesterol and triglyceride transport and is clinically important in blood vessel diseases.

leptin A key hormone of appetite and metabolism.

libido Generally thought of as sexual desire but has psychiatric roots in instinctual energy or what Freud termed the id.

ligaments Bands of cord-like tissue that connect bone to bone.

limbic system A part of the brain that supports a variety of functions including emotion, behavior, and memory. The brain structures of the limbic system include the hippocampus, amygdala, anterior thalamic nuclei, and limbic cortex. The term *limbic* comes from the Latin word *limbus*, meaning border.

Lupus See SLE

Lyme disease A tick-borne infectious illness initially presenting with a headache, fever, fatigue, and a rash called erythema migrans. Long-term consequences of untreated Lyme disease remain controversial.

magnetic resonance imaging A high-resolution imaging technique to see both the structure and function of an organ. In FM, MRI is especially helpful for understanding the brain.

MCS (Multiple Chemical Sensitivities) A chronic, recurring condition caused by the inability to tolerate any one or many of the multiple chemical exposures found in the environment. It appears to be triggered slowly by low level contact with offending chemical substances and can disable those who are severely affected, both at work and in many external situations.

MDD (major depressive disorder) Characterized by pervasive sadness, low mood, and loss of interest in previously enjoyable activities.

metabolites Both the intermediates and products of metabolism.

metastatic Displaced (from the Greek). Usually refers to the spread of disease from one site or organ to another (e.g., cancer metastasis).

mitral valve prolapse (MVP) A heart problem in which the valve that separates the left upper and lower chambers of the heart does not close properly. Sometimes MVP is associated with dysautonomia.

MPS (myofascial pain syndrome) A chronic condition that affects the fascia (connective tissue that covers the muscles). Myofascial pain syndrome may involve either a single muscle or a muscle group. In some cases, the area where a person experiences the pain may not be where the myofascial pain generator is located.

MS (multiple sclerosis) A condition in which the immune system attacks the central nervous system, leading to a loss of normal nerve structure and function.

multidisciplinary approach The decision to use many disciplines to define and apply new ways of understanding complex situations.

myofascial pain Pain in the fascia (connective tissue that covers the muscles).

myopathies Inflammatory and noninflammatory diseases of muscle.

myositis Pathologic inflammation of a muscle.

narcolepsy A neurological disease characterized by excessive daytime sleepiness and nighttime fragmented sleep. It is diagnosed with a sleep study.

National Institutes of Health See NIH

neuralgia Pain produced by a change in neurological structure or function.

neurally mediated hypotension A drop in blood pressure after prolonged motionless standing. It is thought to be one of the dysautonomias.

neurodegenerative disease Any of many diseases in which the nerves no longer communicate effectively with the muscles, often resulting in muscle atrophy or dysfunction.

neuroendocrine Relating to, or involving interaction between, the nervous system and hormones produced by the endocrine glands.

neuropathy A medical term describing disorders of nerves in the peripheral nervous system. Symptoms depend on the type of nerves affected and the body location.

neuropeptide Y A neurotransmitter found in the nervous system that is thought to regulate memory, learning, and metabolism.

neurosensory balance analysis A system for measuring nerve transmission information to and from peripheral extremities and the CNS.

neurotransmitters Body chemicals originating in nerve cells that are used to relay signals.

(NIH) National Institutes of Health A government organization charged with generating high-quality, high-impact medical research.

NK1 A neuroreceptor that works in conjunction with Substance P in the CNS.

NMDA (N-methyl D-aspartate) A water-soluble synthetic substance not normally found in biological tissue.

nociception The unconscious activity produced in the peripheral and central nervous system by stimuli that have the potential to damage tissue. It is not the same as sensing pain, which is a conscious experience.

norepinephrine A chemical messenger that is both a hormone and a neurotransmitter. As a hormone, norepinephrine works on attention and responding actions that are controlled by the brain. It also plays a role in the fight-or-flight response by increasing heart rate, causing the release of glucose, and increasing blood flow.

NSAIDs (Nonsteroidal Anti-Inflammatory Drugs) Prescription and nonprescription medications used to reduce pain, fever and, inflammation. Over-the-counter medications in this category include aspirin, ibuprofen, and naproxen.

off-label Drugs prescribed for any purpose outside the approved indication. Off-label prescribing is legal and commonly practiced.

opiates Drugs in the opiate family are narcotics. In moderate doses they dull the senses, relieve pain, and induce deep sleep, but excessive doses can cause stupor, coma, or convulsions.

orthotics Inserts in shoes that are meant to redistribute weight and correct various medical problems.

osteoarthritis An inflammation that causes joint pain and degeneration. A different disease from rheumatoid arthritis.

PAD (peripheral artery disease) Similar to coronary artery disease but commonly affecting the legs and pelvis.

paresthesia A skin sensation of burning, prickling, itching, or tingling, with no apparent physical cause.

parvovirus A family of very small viruses. Parvovirus B19 causes fifth disease, sometimes called "slapped cheek" disease due to the reddened appearance of the cheeks.

pathophysiological Functional changes associated with symptoms, disorders, diseases, or injuries.

peptic ulcer disease A mucosal lesion in the upper intestinal tract (stomach), often associated with Helicobacter pylori bacterial infection.

perimenopausal The years leading up to menopause, or the cessation of menses (periods).

peripheral neuropathy Damage to the peripheral nervous system that causes a lesion resulting in pain, stinging, numbness, or other discomfort.

phantom limb pain Any sensation in an amputated or missing limb. Phantom pains can occur after any body part has been removed, such as the breast after mastectomy.

pharmacologic The chemical characteristics of drugs.

plantar fasciitis Painful inflammation of the fascia that supports the arches of the foot and heel.

PMR (polymyalgia rheumatica) An inflammatory condition that causes widespread muscle pain and stiffness, particularly in the shoulder girdle and pelvis. Diagnosed with a history, physical exam, and sedimentation rate (blood test).

polymyalgia rheumatica See PMR

postmenopausal The years after menopause (cessation of menses or periods).

precipitator An agent or action that causes something to happen, often prematurely.

progesterone A steroid hormone, essential in the menstrual cycle and pregnancy.

proprioception Feedback of relative body position.

psychosocial The interaction between psychological development and the social environment.

psychosomatic Concerning the mind and body. Sometimes used to indicate bodily symptoms caused by mental or emotional problems.

PTSD (posttraumatic stress disorder) An anxiety disorder that can develop after a terrifying or life-threatening event and is associated with objective neurological changes.

recombinant DNA A form of synthetic DNA. A process that is essential in making certain types of medication such as insulin and growth hormone.

Reynaud's Phenomenon A disorder usually of the hands and feet that results in pain and discoloration and is often triggered by cold temperatures.

rheumatic disease A nonspecific term for medical problems affecting many body organs and locations including heart, bones, joints, kidney, skin, or lung.

rheumatoid arthritis An autoimmune disease causing joint pain and joint deformity and involving multiple organ systems.

RLS (Restless Legs Syndrome) A neurological condition characterized by an irresistible urge to move the legs. Symptoms to induce movement may include creeping, crawling, itching, or gnawing that occur at rest and are relieved with movement.

sedentary Not physically active but settled.

sedimentation rate Also known as erythrocyte sedimentation rate (ESR), it is the rate at which blood precipitates in one hour. ESR is elevated in many inflammatory diseases such as polymyalgia rheumatica.

sensory pathways Regions of the body that detect touch, pain pressure, temperature, and body position (proprioception).

serotonin A neurotransmitter that regulates sleep patterns, mood, a feeling of well-being, and inhibition of pain, it is also a vasoconstrictor in the brain, blood, and gut.

Sjögren's Syndrome An autoimmune disease in which the white blood cells "attack" the glands in the eyes, nose, mouth, and other mucous members, making these areas dry and uncomfortable. It is also associated with fatigue.

SLE (systemic lupus erythematosus) A chronic inflammatory autoimmune disorder affecting any one or more of the following: skin, joints, blood cells, kidneys, heart, lungs.

sleep apnea Disordered breathing that can be obstructive, central, or mixed. Associated with alternating snores and pauses without breathing.

slow-wave sleep Deep stages 3 and 4 nonrapid eye movement sleep. Eighty percent of growth hormone is made during deep sleep.

SNRIs (serotonin norepinephrine reuptake inhibitors) A type of antidepressant that acts on both serotonin and norepinephrine levels.

somatosensory cortex The main sensory receptive area in the cortex of the brain.

spatial navigation The ability to move accurately between elements or objects that one can sense.

sphygmomanometer Medical device used for determining blood pressure.

SSRIs (Selective Serotonin Reuptake Inhibitors) A type of antidepressant that acts on serotonin levels such as Zoloft and Prozac.

stage-4 sleep Stages 3 and 4 sleep are considered deep sleep, with Stage-4 being the most intense and characterized in sleep studies by rhythmic delta waves.

statin Technically, statins are MHG-CoA reductase inhibitors and refer to a class of medications that lower blood lipid levels and thereby the risk of blood vessel diseases.

statin intolerance Muscle pain or perceived weakness in persons on a statin medication but no laboratory signs of muscle damage. May occur in 5 to10 percent of persons on statins and may be relieved by changing statins.

stenosis A narrowing. In medical terminology, stenosis usually refers to an abnormal narrowing of a blood vessel or a tubular structure like the bile duct or the intestinal track.

steroid Naturally occurring hormones including sex steroids: estrogen, progesterone, testosterone, and corticosteroids, and including glucocorticoids, mineralcorticoids, and cortisol

Substance P A neuropeptide considered a key transmitter of pain to the brain.

suprapubic Structures located above the pubic bone.

syndrome A term used in the understanding of an illness when the underlying abnormalities are not as well understood.

synovitis An abnormal fluid collection around joints.

synovium Tissue that surrounds and nourishes and lubricates the joints.

symptomatic diverticulitis A common digestive ailment that is associated with the formation of pouches in the colon. Symptoms include lower abdominal pain and fever.

tender point A painful sensation felt when pressure is applied to a specific, localized location.

Tender Point Survey The current "gold-standard" exam used to diagnose FM when widespread pain is present. There are eighteen designated tender points used to diagnose FM. During diagnosis, 4 kg of force is exerted at each of the eighteen points; the patient must feel pain at eleven or more of these points for fibromyalgia to be diagnosed. Four kg of force is about the amount of pressure required to blanch the thumbnail.

tendonitis Inflammation of a tendon. A tendon is a tough fibrous tissue that is meant to be flexible and connects muscle to bone. Inflammation results in pain.

TENS (transcutaneous electrical nerve stimulator) Used to apply electrical current through the skin for pain control.

testosterone An androgen steroid produced by the testes (large quantities) or the ovaries (small quantities).

theory An explanation to a set of observations that explains a body of facts and the laws they are based upon.

third-party payers Typically medical insurance companies.

thyroid An endocrine gland in the neck that produces thyroid hormone and is essential for life.

tilt table test A medical procedure used to diagnose one of the dysautonomias. It involves serial blood pressure monitoring during prolonged motionless standing in a table that slowly tilts.

TMD (Temporomandibular Joint Dysfunction) A disorder that affects the functioning of the jawbone area but also includes the muscles and cartilage throughout the face, head, and neck. Symptoms can range from headaches to a painfully immobile jaw.

TMS (Tension Myositis Syndrome) The theory that untreatable pain functions as an unconscious distraction from dangerous emotions and when emotions are surfaced, pain disappears.

transmucosal Across or through a mucous membrane. Many drugs are administered transmucosally.

trigger point Hyperirritable skeletal muscle knots or areas that are associated with palpable taut band changes in the muscle. When compressed a trigger point may hurt locally or send pain to another nearby region of the body (referred pain).

trochanter A portion of the thigh bone. In FM a bursea located near the greater trochanter may become inflamed and painful (tronchateric bursitis).

tryptophan An amino acid necessary for normal growth in infants and for nitrogen balance in adults. The body cannot produce it; it must be obtained from the diet.

ultrasound therapy High-frequency sound waves that produce heat and may relieve pain. Often used by physical therapists.

unipolar disease See MDD

vasculitis Inflammation in the blood vessels.

vestibular Relating to the inner ear.

virus A microscopic infectious agent unable to reproduce without a host.

vulvar vestibulitis Redness and pain in a specific region of the female genitalia.

vulvodynia Literally meaning pain in the external female genitalia. Vulvodynia may include burning and irritation and result in difficulty sitting or having sexual intercourse.

Bibliography

Armstrong, D. J., G. K. Meenagh, I. Bickle, A. S. Lee, E. S. Curran, and M. B. Finch. 2006. Vitamin D deficiency is associated with anxiety and depression in fibromyalgia. *Clinical Rheumatology* 26–4:551–554.

Arnold, L. D., G. A. Bachmann, R. Rosen, S. Kelly, and G. G. Rhoads. 2006. Vulvodynia: Characteristics and associations with comorbidities and quality of life. *Obstetrics and Gynecology* 107–3:617–624.

Baldry, Peter. *Myofascial Pain and Fibromyalgia Syndromes: A Clinical Guide to Diagnosis and Management.* London: Churchill Livingstone, 2001.

Bandura, A. 1977. Self-efficacy: Toward a unifying theory of behavior change. *Psychological Review* 84:191–215.

Bennett, R., S. R. Clark, L. Goldberg, et al. 1989. Aerobic fitness in patients with fibrositis. *Arthritis and Rheumatism* 32:454–460.

Bennett, R. 1999. Emerging concepts in the neurobiology of chronic pain: Evidence of abnormal sensory processing in fibromyalgia. *Mayo Clinic Proceedings* 74:385–398.

Bennett, R. M., S. C. Clark, and J. Walczyk. 1998. A randomized, double-blind, placebo-controlled study of growth hormone in the treatment of fibromyalgia. *American Journal of Medicine* 104–3:227–231.

Bennett, R. M. 2002. Rational management of fibromyalgia. *Rheumatic Diseases Clinics of North America Journal* May 28–2:xiii–xixv.

Bennett, Robert. 2008. *Understanding Pain.* [online, 2008] Fibromyalgia Information Foundation Web site. http://www.myalgia.com.

Bigelow, Stacy L. *Fibromyalgia: Simple Relief through Movement.* New York City, NY: John Wiley & Sons, Inc., 2000.

Blehm, R. 2006. Physical therapy and other nonpharmacologic approaches to fibromyalgia management. *Current Pain and Headache Reports* 10–5:333–338.

Buckelew, S. P., R. Conway, J. Parker, et al. 1998. Biofeedback/relaxation training and exercise interventions for fibromyalgia: A prospective trial. *Arthritis Care and Research* 11:196–209.

Burckhardt, C. S., and K. D. Jones. 2003. Adult measures of pain: The McGill Pain Questionnaire (MPQ), Rheumatoid Arthritis Pain Scale (RAPS), Short-Form McGill Pain Questionnaire (SF-MPQ), Verbal Descriptive Scale (VDS), Visual Analog Scale (VAS), and West Haven-Yale Multidisciplinary Pain Inventory (WHYMPI). *Arthritis Care and Research* 49–5S:S96–S104.

Buskila, D., P. Sarzi-Puttini, and J. N. Ablin. 2007. The genetics of fibromyalgia syndrome. *Pharmacogenomics* 8–1:67–74.

Clark, S. R., K. D. Jones, C. S. Burckhardt, et al. 2001. Exercise for patients with fibromyalgia: Risks versus benefits. *Current Rheumatology Reports* 3:135–146.

Cohen, H., L. Neumann, Y. Haiman, M. A. Matar, J. Press, and D. Buskila. 2002. Prevalence of post-traumatic stress disorder in fibromyalgia patients: Overlapping syndromes or post-traumatic fibromyalgia syndrome? *Seminars in Arthritis and Rheumatism* 32–1:38–50.

Crooks, V. A. 2007. Exploring the altered daily geographies and lifeworlds of women living with fibromyalgia syndrome: A mixed-method approach. *Social Science and Medicine* 64–3:577–588.

Farhi, Donna. *The Breathing Book: Good Health and Vitality through Essential Breath Work.* New York: Henry Holt, 2007.

Hadhazy, V. A., J. Ezzo, P. Creamer, et al. 2000. Mind-body therapies for the treatment of fibromyalgia. A systematic review. *Journal of Rheumatology* 27:2911–2918.

Hakkinen, A., K. Hakkinene, P. Hannonen, et al. 2001. Strength training induced adaptations in neuromuscular function of premenopausal women with fibromyalgia: Comparison with healthy women. *Annals of the Rheumatic Diseases* 60:21–26.

Hammond, William A. *Spinal Irritation.* New York: D Appleton and Company, 1886.

Holman, A. J., R. A. Neiman, and R. E. Ettlinger. 2002. Pramipexole for fibromyalgia: The first open label, multicenter experience. *Arthritis and Rheumatism* 46–9:S106.

Hooper, M. M., T. A. Stellato, P. T. Hallowell, B. A. Seitz, and R. W. Moskowitz. 2007. Musculoskeletal findings in obese subjects before and after weight loss following bariatric surgery. *International Journal of Obesity (London)* 31–1:114–120.

Jones, C. J., K. D. Jones, D. N. Rutledge, L. Matallana, and D. Rooks. 2008. Self-assessed physical function levels of women with fibromyalgia: A national survey. *Women's Health Issues* 18(5): 406–412.

Jones, K. D., and D. G. Adams. 2005. How to diagnose and treat fibromyalgia. *Arthritis Practitioner* 1–3:14–20.

Jones, K. D., C. S. Burckhardt, S. R. Clark, et al. 2002. A randomized controlled trial of muscle strengthening versus flexibility training in fibromyalgia. *Journal of Rheumatology* 29:1041–1048.

Jones, K. D., C. S. Burckhardt, N. A. Perrin, G. Hanson, A. A. Deodhar, and R. M. Bennett. 2007. Growth hormone response to acute exercise normalizes with long-term pyridostigmine but does not change IGF-1. *Journal of Rheumatology* 34–4: 1103–1111.

Jones, K. D., P. Deodhar, A. Lorentzen, R. M. Bennett, and A. A. Deodhar. 2007. Growth hormone perturbations in fibromyalgia: A review. *Seminars in Arthritis and Rheumatism* 36–6:357–379.

Jones, K. D., and J. H. Hoffman. 2006. Exercise in chronic pain: Opening the therapeutic window. *International Journal of Active Aging* 4:1–9.

Jones, K. D., J. H. Hoffman, and D. G. Adams. "Exercise and fibromyalgia." In *Understanding Fitness: How Exercise Fuels Health and Fight Disease*, edited by Julie K. Silver and Christopher Morin. Westport, CT: Praeger Press, 2008, 170–181.

Jones, K. D., F. Horak, K. S. Winters, and R. M. Bennett. 2009. Fibromyalgia is associated with impaired balance and falls. *Journal of Clinical Rheumatology* 15–1:16–21.

Jones, K. D., C. R. Shillam, R. L. Ross, and D. G. Adams. 2007. Fibromyalgia in older adults: A guide for rational management. *Practical Pain Management* 7–1:68–72.

Karaaslan, Y., S. Haznedaroglu, and M. Ozturk. 2000. Joint hypermobility and primary fibromyalgia: a clinical enigma. *Journal of Rheumatology* 27:1774–1776.

Kasper, S., and E. Resinger. 2001. Panic disorder: The place of benzodiazepines and selective serotonin reuptake inhibitors. *European Neuropsychopharmacology* 11–4:307–321.

Katon, W., M. Sullivan, and E. Walker. 2001. Medical symptoms without identified pathology: Relationship to psychiatric disorders, childhood and adult trauma, and personality traits. *Annals of Internal Medicine* 134–Pt 2:917–925.

Kindler, L. L., K. D. Jones, and K. Holton. 2009 (in press, invited). Dietary interventions in fibromyalgia: Past reports, future directions. *Rheumatic Disease Clinics of North America*.

Lorig, K., R. L. Chastain, E. Ung, et al. 1989. Development and valuation of a scale to measure perceived self-efficacy in people with arthritis. *Arthritis and Rheumatism* 32:37–44.

Marek, Claudia C. *The First Year—Fibromyalgia: An Essential Guide for the Newly Diagnosed.* New York: Marlowe and Company, 2003.

McCain, G., D. A. Bell, F. M. Mai, et al. 1988. A controlled study of the effects of a supervised cardiovascular fitness training program on the manifestations of primary fibromyalgia. *Arthritis and Rheumatism* 31:1135–1141.

Metts, J. F. 2001. Interstitial cystitis: Urgency and frequency syndrome. *American Family Physician* 64–7:1199–1206.

Moldofsky, H., P. Scarisbrick, R. England, et al. 1975. Musculoskeletal symptoms and nonREM sleep disturbance in patients with fibrositis syndrome and healthy subjects. *Psychosomatic Medicine* 34:341–351.

Moldofsky, H. 2002. Management of sleep disorders in fibromyalgia. *Rheumatic Disease Clinics of North America* 28–2: 353–365.

Nicassio, P. M., E. G. Moxham, C. E. Schuman, and R. N. Gevirtz. 2002. The contribution of pain, reported sleep quality, and depressive symptoms to fatigue in fibromyalgia. *Clinical Journal of Pain* 100–3:271–279.

O'Malley, P. G., E. Balden, G. Tomkins, J. Santoro, K. Kroenke, J. L. Jackson. 2000. Treatment of fibromyalgia with antidepressants: A meta-analysis. *Journal of General Internal Medicine* 15–9:659–666.

Otis, John. *Managing Chronic Pain. A Cognitive—Behavioral Therapy Approach Workbook.* New York: Oxford Press, 2007.

Penrod, J. R., S. Bernatsky, V. Adam, M. Baron, N. Dayan, and P. L. Dobkin. 2004. Health services costs and their determinants in women with fibromyalgia. *Journal of Rheumatology* Jul 31:1391–1398.

Pierrynowski, M. R., P. M. Tiidus, and V. Galea. 2005. Women with fibromyalgia walk with an altered muscle synergy. *Gait and Posture* Nov 22–3:210–218.

Plesh, O., D. Curtis, J. Levine, W. D. McCall Jr. 2000. Amitriptyline treatment of chronic pain in patients with temporomandibular disorders. *Journal of Oral Rehabilitation* 27–10:834–841.

Rossy, L. A., S. P. Buckelew, N. Dorr, et al. 1999. A meta-analysis of fibromyalgia treatment interventions. *Annals of Behavioral Medicine* 21:180–191.

Russell, I. J., and K. G. Raphael. 2008. Fibromyalgia syndrome: Presentation, diagnosis, differential diagnosis, and vulnerability. *CNS Spectrums* 3–S5:6–11.

Russell, I. J. 2008. Fibromyalgia syndrome: approach to management. *CNS Spectrums* 3–S5:27–33.

Russell, I. J. 2008. Fibromyalgia syndrome: New developments in pathophysiology and management. Introduction. *CNS Spectrums* 3–S5:4–5.

Sherman, J. J., D. C. Turk, and A. Okifuji. 2000. Prevalence and impact of posttraumatic stress disorder-like symptoms on patients with fibromyalgia syndrome. *The Clinical Journal of Pain* 16–2:127–134.

Sim, J., and N. Adams. 2002. Systematic review of randomized controlled trials of nonpharmacological interventions for fibromyalgia. *The Clinical Journal of Pain* 18:324–336.

Staud, R., and M. L. Smitherman. 2002. Peripheral and central sensitization in fibromyalgia: Pathogenetic role. *Current Pain Headache and Reports* 6–4:259–266.

Staud, R. 2006. Biology and therapy of fibromyalgia: pain in fibromyalgia syndrome. *Arthritis Research and Therapy* 8–3:208.

Trock, David H., and Francis Chamberlain. *Healing Fibromyalgia. The Three Step Solution*. New Jersey: John Wiley & Sons, 2007.

Turk, Dennis C., and Frits Winter. *The Pain Survival Guide: How to Reclaim Your Life*. Washington, D.C.: American Psychological Association Press, 2006.

Valim, V., L. M. Oliveira, A. Suda, et al. 2002. Peak oxygen uptake and ventilatory anaerobic threshold in fibromyalgia. *Journal of Rheumatology* 29:353–357.

Van Santen, M., P. Bolwijn, R. Landewe, et al. 2002 High or low intensity aerobic fitness training in fibromyalgia: Does it matter? *Journal of Rheumatology* 29:582–587.

Wigers, S. H., T. C. Stiles, and P. A. Vogel. 1996. Effects of aerobic exercise versus stress management treatment in fibromyalgia: A 4.5 year prospective study. *Scandinavian Journal of Rheumatology* 25:77–86.

Williams, D. A., and R. H. Gracely. 2007. Biology and therapy of fibromyalgia. Functional magnetic resonance imaging findings in fibromyalgia. *Arthritis Research and Therapy* 8–6:224.

Wolfe, F., J. Anderson, D. Harkness, R. M. Bennett, X. J. Caro, D. L. Goldenberg, et al. 1997. A prospective, longitudinal, multicenter study of service utilization and costs in fibromyalgia. *Arthritis and Rheumatism* 40–9:1560–1570.

Wolfe, F., H. A, Smythe, M. B. Yunus, et al. 1990. The American College of Rheumatology 1990 criteria for the classification of fibromyalgia. *Arthritis and Rheumatism* 33:160–172.

Wood, P. B., J. C. Patterson, J. J. Sunderland, K. H. Tainter, M. F. Glabus, and D. L. Lilien. 2007. Reduced presynaptic dopamine activity in fibromyalgia syndrome demonstrated with positron emission tomography: A pilot study. *The Clinical Journal of Pain* 8–1:51–58.

ONLINE RESOURCES:

Advocates for Fibromyalgia Funding, Treatment, Education, and Research: www.affter.org
American College of Rheumatology: www.rheumatology.org
Arthritis Foundation: www.arthritis.org
Fibromyalgia Association Created for Education and Self-Help (FACES): www.fibro-cop.org
Fibromyalgia Information Foundation: www.myalgia.com
Fibromyalgia Network: www.fmnetnews.com
FM/CFS Canada: www.fm-cfs.ca
National Center for Complementary and Alternative Medicine: www.nccam.nih.gov
National Fibromyalgia Association: www.fmaware.org
National Fibromyalgia Partnership, Inc.: www.fmpartnership.org
National Institute of Arthritis, Musculoskeletal, and Skin Diseases: www.niams.nih.gov
Social Security Administration: www.ssa.gov/disability
The Fibromyalgia Connection: www.fmah.org

Index

Note: Entries with page numbers followed by an f refer to illustrations on the designated page.

About the Authors

Kim Dupree Jones, RN, FNP, PhD, is an associate professor of nursing and assistant professor of medicine at Oregon Health and Science University in Portland, Oregon. Her undergraduate nursing degree is from the University of Tennessee, her master and nurse practitioner degrees from Emory University in Atlanta, Georgia, and her PhD from Oregon Health and Science University. Her area of expertise is exercise physiology and neuroendocrinology in fibromyalgia. She has been the principal investigator on five major research studies funded by National Institutes of Health, Industry, and Foundations and a co-investigator on twenty-five–plus fibromyalgia research studies, mostly in collaboration with colleagues on the Oregon Fibromyalgia Research and Treatment Team. She has written more than 100 publications and is a frequently invited international speaker for patients, clinicians, and researchers investigating fibromyalgia. She maintains a fibromyalgia clinical practice at Oregon Health and Science University and is current president of the Fibromyalgia Information Foundation (FIF).

Janice Holt Hoffman, CES, is a certified clinical exercise specialist with advanced training in working with special populations. She has presented workshops throughout the western United States for the American Council on Exercise that are designed to prepare upcoming fitness leaders for their certification exams and help current fitness professionals develop quality leadership skills. For the past nine years, she has been involved in clinical research studies at Oregon Health and Science University in Portland, Oregon, working as project director for the Oregon Fibromyalgia Research and Treatment Team on research drug trials. She has led the exercise component in a variety of exercise-based research studies, including fibromyalgia research and breast cancer survivorship research, and has choreographed six special population exercise workout DVDs. She serves on the board of the Fibromyalgia Information Foundation (FIF).